W9-BXL-742

EMBRACING THE WOLF

EMBRACING THE WOLF

A Lupus Victim and Her Family Learn to Live with Chronic Disease

Joanna Baumer Permut

Cherokee Publishing Company
Atlanta, Georgia
1989

Library of Congress Cataloging-in-Publication Data

Permut, Joanna Baumer.
  Embracing the wolf/by Joanna Baumer Permut.
    p. cm.
  Bibliography: p.
  ISBN 0-87797-166-8
  1. Permut, Joanna Baumer—Health.   2. Systemic lupus
erythematosus—Patients—United States—Biography.   3. Systemic
lupus erythematosus—Patients—Family relationships.   4. Systemic
lupus erythematosus—Psychological aspects.   I. Title.
RC924.5.L85P43   1989
362.1'9677—dc19
[B]   88-9193
                                                                                                    CIP

This book is printed on acid-free paper which conforms to the American National
Standard Z39.48-1984 *Permanence of Paper for Printed Library Materials.* Paper that
conforms to this standard's requirements for pH, alkaline reserve and freedom from
groundwood is anticipated to last several hundred years without significant deteriora-
tion under normal library use and storage conditions. ⊗

Manufactured in the United States of America

First Edition

ISBN: 0-87797-166-8

98 97 96 95 94 93 92 91 90 89   10 9 8 7 6 5 5 3 2

Edited by Alexa Selph

Design by Paulette Lambert

Cherokee Publishing Company is an operating division of
the Larlin Corporation, PO Box 1730, Marietta, Georgia 30061

For Steven, my ballast,
who gives me support in the darkness of disease

and

For Peggy, my mother
1915–1982
who gave me the strength and spirit to endure

Contents

The young take good health for granted. Even the rest of us, no longer young, expect to be well until a ripe old age. Disability is something that happens to others. Illness is something temporary, a minor setback, and hopefully will either go away by itself or be healed by modern medicines. We are never prepared to be chronically sick.

Thus, when an incurable illness unexpectedly strikes, the effects can be devastating to patients as well as to their families and friends. The response may depend, in part, on the severity of the disease. Paradoxically, patients and their relatives sometimes adapt better to catastrophic medical problems than to equally serious but less obvious conditions. For example, a young man in an automobile accident who suffers a broken neck and is paralyzed from the neck down receives immediate sympathy. Despite the enormity of the problem, there is generally a set of support systems to deal with this permanent injury. Families find the inner strength to help such patients, despite the fact that tremendous adjustments are necessary. We are somehow able to adapt to awful medical tragedies.

On the other hand, patients with less overt disease, which may express itself with more subtle symptoms, frequently receive little sympathy, and may even have trouble convincing family members that anything is truly wrong. It is as if it is easier for us to be more tolerant of paralysis than of a spouse who complains constantly of fatigue. We can see an amputated leg and understand clearly its meaning, but a patient with aching joints who can no longer run or open jars may not be taken seriously. It is tempting for us to assume that patients who do not appear ill and who have only subjective symptoms can simply "get hold of themselves" and conquer their complaints by sheer will power. No one expects that of a patient with advanced cancer or with a severe stroke.

A disease such as systemic lupus erythematosus is often insidious and subtle in onset. Many of the symptoms are subjective, such as fatigue, joint aches, or a general feeling of being ill.

When such symptoms develop in a young, vigorous mother, it is understandable that her healthy, active husband might find it difficult to comprehend why his wife can no longer keep up with him. It is especially frightening for him that there are no definite, objective signs of disease. He hears the complaints but cannot understand their nature. Some are so vague as to suggest a possible psychosomatic origin to him.

Even physicians may be skeptical of nonspecific complaints and overlook the possibility of an underlying serious disorder. After all, there are many people who are exhausted most of the time and who have multiple aches and pains that have no recognizable organic basis. Lupus cannot be suspected in all of them.

In this book, Joanna Permut focuses on her relationship with her husband as he at first confuses her symptoms with emotional illness and then later makes a major effort to understand the unusual disorder affecting his wife. She graphically chronicles her own deep fears and her desperate need for others to understand all of her symptoms in the context of lupus. Joanna also emphasizes the importance of establishing a good relationship with her physicians as they struggle with not only the diagnosis and treatment, but also the emotional aspects of her illness.

Joanna Permut shows that one should not and cannot fight a chronic illness alone. Her story should be of enormous help to all young families who are coping with persistent illness. Open communication between husband and wife, between patient and physician, seems to be the best medicine of all.

—Robert H. Gifford, M.D.
Associate Dean for Education
and Student Affairs, Yale
University School of Medicine

*Disease may score a direct hit on only one member of
a family, but shrapnel tears the flesh of the others.*
—*Betty Rollin*

Over the years I have read many books written by patients suffering from chronic disease. Their stories, though compelling and absorbing, sometimes leave me dissatisfied for the reason that too often they neglect to mention the adverse affects of their diseases on their healthy spouses. Granted, many spouses may prefer not to have their difficulties described in black and white. But I also think that too many patients are so self-absorbed with their own overwhelming problems—physical, emotional, and psychological—that it may not even occur to them that their mates are riddled with an entirely different set of complaints.

The chronically ill need all the support they can rally to face the consequences of disease. It is only natural to expect understanding and solace from your husband or wife. But too often when the patient turns to her healthy spouse for help, she instead finds him preoccupied with his own fears and frustrations. While it is true that spouses do not feel the symptoms and pain of disease, they nevertheless suffer, despair, and worry. If the pressure of caring for a chronically ill patient becomes too burdensome, some spouses may actually disappear, develop physical problems of their own, lose their jobs, or suffer breakdowns. They may turn to alcohol or drug abuse to comfort them, to protect them from the stark realities of life at home with a sick mate. Many times, in searching for a pillar of support, the patient instead finds a normal human being, terrified, in conflict, and at a total loss to cope with either his mate or the many ramifications of the disease.

Healthy spouses cannot and should not be ignored. And who better than we, the chronically ill, to address our spouses' myriad problems? Who better than we to flush their negative emotions and overwhelming fears into the open so they may be tended and repaired? In so doing we deliver ourselves from the depths of self-preoccupation at the same time that we restore hope and spirit to our mates. If we recognize the needs of our spouses, they can then become that pillar of support we so urgently require in order to survive the onslaught of chronic disease.

Because I have lived with systemic lupus for a decade, I can bear witness to the toll it has taken on my husband as I have watched him struggle to accept my illness and wrestle with his own emotions. When one partner in a marriage is afflicted with a chronic disease, it not only affects the patient but intrudes upon the entire family, drastically influencing the dynamics of the marriage and disrupting the peace and serenity of the healthy spouse. It often affects the children as well, but in varying degrees, depending on their ages, their relationships with their parents, the stability of life at home, and the severity of the disease. I feel the story of chronic disease can be fully told only if it includes the patient, the spouse, and the children, with emphasis on the patient and spouse as a couple.

It is especially difficult to be sick in today's society, where illness is taboo and health is *in*, where so much emphasis is placed on nutrition, exercise, and keeping fit, where advertising would have you believe that all you need to do to be well is to ingest certain products that miraculously eradicate problems ranging from wrinkles to heart disease. Perhaps the most difficult facet of chronic illness is that both patient and spouse know it has moved in to stay. Because it is chronic, it will live as long as the patient lives. Maggie Strong, in her book *Mainstay*, provides the most chilling, yet accurate, description of chronic disease that I have ever read: "Chronic illnesses don't always kill, or not for decades. They limit and disable. They blind. They bring pain. They threaten adulthood and sexuality. They age, robbing the sickest of energy for anything but biological functioning. They paralyze and leave the brain alert or they snuff out memory and logic and leave the body robust. But they don't go away."

In this narrative I have not dwelled on my physical problems with lupus, except to set the stage; in my case they do not constitute the greatest difficulty of lupus. Rather, the *psychological* effects of lupus on me as the patient, next on my husband, and most important on us as partners in life, have often been devastating and overwhelming. For Steven and me, fighting lupus psychologically is still the hardest battle of all, for it is a perpetual challenge to our spirits.

Lupus is a particularly difficult disease to cope with, primarily due to its unpredictable nature and its wide-ranging symptoms. When lupus flares, the patient is caught unaware. Seldom does she know when she will be attacked or what part of her body will be involved. Never does she know how long the flare-up will last. As a result, she does not know to what extent or for how long she will have to curtail her activities. It could be days, weeks, or months. Lupus could keep her in bed at home, or hospitalize her. She may suffer from only a fever and aching muscles, or she may experience serious organ involvement of the brain, heart, lungs, or kidneys. The lupus patient may feel entirely well one morning, and by noon be too weak to move her limbs. Stiff joints may make it impossible for her to get out of bed when she wakens, but by nightfall she may feel lively again. Quite often she must live with a good deal of pain, as well as with drugs, doctors, and examinations. Never does she completely understand what is happening within her own body.

This is Steven's and my story of learning to live with lupus during the crucial years when we passed through many difficult stages until we finally reached acceptance. Hard as it was, sometimes nearly impossible, we were at last willing and able to rearrange our lives to accommodate lupus, to embrace it into our family, to make peace with the enemy. It is my hope that by sharing our story, other lupus patients and their spouses, as well as victims of other chronic diseases and their partners, may gain some insight from our experience. At the very least, it may reassure them to know that they are not alone in their fight for survival.

* * * * * * * *

Since the inception of this book, many people have offered their ideas, support, and encouragement. I am indebted to them all.

I wish to thank my close, caring friends for their interest in my project and their unflinching belief in me. When I was afflicted by "writer's block" or discouraged by rejection slips, they injected me with the drive to proceed, and at all costs to keep on writing.

Very special appreciation goes to Ed and Rhoda Tripp and Katrina Van Tassel, who read the manuscript not once but several times and, from the beginning, urged me to continue. I am especially grateful for their editorial expertise and guidance through the last critical stages of the book. Most important, I have been blessed with an insightful, keen editor, Alexa Selph, who somehow managed to be firm yet flexible simultaneously, and an enthusiastic, progressive publisher, Ken Boyd, who demonstrated a personal interest in the book, lupus, and me, since the day he accepted the manuscript. Working with both has been a rewarding experience.

I also want to thank my doctors for contributing in one way or another to this book. In particular, Dr. Robert H. Gifford and Dr. David B. Melchinger deserve special mention. Both have been my physicians as well as my friends throughout the trying course of lupus. Their understanding of me, my disease, and my family life has been sustaining in its endurance. They are to be especially credited for their ongoing attempts to improve my health and my attitude, and for standing by me through my most difficult moments. As for this book, both doctors were active participants from the start, as they spent a great deal of time talking with me about my ideas and contributing their own. Special thanks go to Dr. Gifford for writing the Foreword and the description of lupus in the Appendix, and to Dr. Melchinger for producing a glossary of medical terms.

Words cannot possibly express enough gratitude to my husband, Steven, and to my daughter, Lisa. Both provided moral support and unflagging encouragement and nourishment. They listened intently as I unraveled my thoughts, they made worthy suggestions, and from the beginning, they believed in my cause.

In particular, Steven deserves praise—first for his determination to come to an understanding of lupus, and second, for his courage in allowing me to write about some of the most intimate episodes in our marriage.

CHAPTER ONE

The Wolf Stalks His Prey

As they close the gap between themselves and their prey, the wolves become excited but remain restrained. They quicken their paces, wag their tails, and peer ahead intently. . . . This stage of the hunt is the stalk.
—*L. David Mech*

In July of 1976 my husband, daughter, and I returned to the United States after living in Brussels for two years. Steven had accepted an assistant professorship at Yale University's School of Organization and Management in New Haven. Although we regretted leaving Belgium, we were nevertheless excited to come to Yale. For Steven it was an honor to be asked to join a prestigious faculty and to help design the first core marketing curriculum at a new business school. For me it was a return to familiar territory, where I had spent my childhood years and attended school. It was the home of family and friends. It was also where Steven and I had met and fallen in love. We rented a small house in the Connecticut shoreline town of Guilford, a block from Long Island Sound. Steven started teaching, and Lisa began second grade in the nearby elementary school.

In Belgium I had worked as Steven's editor and secretary. Steven taught marketing in Boston University's overseas MBA program and together we worked on consulting assignments. I found this a very rewarding time that cemented us during our first years of marriage. When we returned to Yale, the university seemed a logical place to look for work, since I had previously been employed there. I quickly found a job in the administration, operating out of Woodbridge Hall, the hub of university activity.

The years in Belgium and the ensuing time at Yale were the happiest years of my life. Lisa was well settled, making good friends, and enjoying school. Besides playing the piano, she had taken up the violin and was a member of her school orchestra. Steven enjoyed teaching and maintained an active consulting practice as well. I was proud to be a working woman with a "mini-career," as I liked to call it, and prouder still to be contributing to our family income.

We eventually bought our own house in the woods of Guilford. With a full-time job I rose at six, prepared breakfast and saw Lisa off to school, drove half an hour to New Haven with Steven, worked all day, and sometimes even managed to swim at the gym during my lunch hour. We were usually home by six, where Lisa and her after-school babysitter, Kim, greeted us. Then I would make dinner and endeavor to be a lively mother and wife. I was diligent about devoting my remaining energy of the day to my family. There was never any question in my mind about priorities. Family was first. Job was second. I helped Lisa with piano, took turns with Steven assisting her with homework and reading to her at bedtime. Steven and I spent an hour or two alone after Lisa was asleep. I was exhausted, but felt complete and fulfilled. Our weekends were necessarily occupied with errands, housecleaning, and entertaining guests. But we also packed in a lot of family fun at football and hockey games, theater, concerts, and occasional day trips to New York City.

The business of life was moving along. Since I had been an avid horseback rider as a child, I thought it was important to start Lisa right away. We often rode together and enjoyed sharing this special activity. All three of us spent our summers swimming, boating, and vacationing around New England when our jobs permitted. When Lisa was nine, she began overnight camp in Maine. In the winter we occasionally went skiing, though I did not participate. I never wanted to ski because the cold and heights always bothered me. Lisa, however, was a quick learner, soon able to accompany Steven down the slopes, while I spent my days back

4

at the inn, safe and warm, reading. Steven and I always made time to be alone together too. My parents were happy to take care of their only grandchild. This allowed us an infrequent short weekend to get reacquainted, to enjoy a few romantic days and nights together.

My job in the Office of the Secretary was personally rewarding. My boss was easy to work with, kind, and relaxed. As his administrative assistant, my primary responsibility involved managing the Honorary Degrees Program. In this capacity I dealt with some famous and interesting people. I remember those days when I was so intoxicated with happiness that I wondered if it would last.

I had already faced enough adversity in my life to know that no one can live in such a harmonious state forever. I had lost my older sister and only sibling, Connie, to cancer when she was twenty-four. At the time I was nineteen. Her death devastated me, for we were very close. Unfortunately I had not been told how seriously ill she was. I could neither understand nor accept her death. Instead, I raged at it. Connie's death affected my mother, in particular, very adversely. She felt guilty, as if in some way she were responsible for her firstborn's cancer, and she mourned in her own private way. Retreating to her bedroom for days at a stretch, she was unable to communicate with anyone. Those times were extremely hard on me, as I was powerless to do anything to alleviate her grief. I, as the only child now, felt a compelling responsibility to make my mother happy again. My mother and I lost whatever small amount of faith we had in God when Connie died. It might have been easier for us both if we had had some sort of religious belief to sustain us. Instead we muddled through in a state of anger and excruciating, self-flagellating grief.

Two years after Connie's death I nearly lost my mother to colon cancer, but she recovered miraculously. Nevertheless, it was a traumatic experience that again put me on the edge of death with a loved one. Then there were the stormy years of my first divorce, which brought more stress and anxiety, and which signified yet another loss.

Because of these past troubles, I had a premonition that my present life was too satisfactory, that something dark and heavy would arrive, be it financial problems, marital trauma, whatever. But the last thing I suspected, at my young age of twenty-nine, was disease.

****

During the autumn of 1977 I was plagued with symptoms that I did not understand. Mostly, I was exhausted all the time. I survived until noon on overdoses of coffee, then slept during my lunch hour on the sofa in my office, barely making it to five o'clock on still more caffeine. I dozed in the car and, when I arrived home, was unable to make dinner or cope with Lisa. I had to lie down and be still. Steven took over in many capacities ungrudgingly, especially with Lisa. He had been her father since she was five and was natural and relaxed with her. They enjoyed a unique, close relationship. Kim continued her duties as babysitter and began to help with the cleaning too. Soon it was also necessary for her to cook most of our meals. Not only was I exhausted, despite long sleeps and naps, I also ached all over, particularly in my joints. Several times I had so much pain in my hands that I could not lift a dinner plate, cut my meat, or shift gears in my car. I had hot flashes and, when I took my temperature, discovered that I had a slight fever of about a degree and a half. I was breathless even when I was not overexerting myself. On staircases I became so short of breath that I had to stop in the middle, rest, and wait to regain my breath before I climbed to the top. I had a continually sore throat that felt as if a fire were burning deep down in my chest, shooting its flames up into my throat, and I lost six pounds. I was always very cold, and the tips of my fingers often turned a ghastly white.

After feeling this way for a few weeks, I finally went to see my internist. In fact, I saw Dr. Jones* several times over a period

*fictitious name

of three months, complaining of these symptoms. He tested me for things like anemia and thyroid dysfunction. He discovered mild anemia, for which he prescribed iron pills, and a slightly low white-blood count. Neither of these findings alarmed him. He usually sent me home saying, "You probably just have a low-grade virus." I was getting impatient with Dr. Jones's queries about the state of my marriage, finances, child, and job. The implication was clear: he thought I was either a hypochondriac or "emotionally unhappy," to use his words. In fact, I was neither.

My "virus" persisted. After I became so weak and tired I could not go to work for a while, I finally told Dr. Jones that, if he could not find out what my problem was, my husband was going to take me to the Mayo Clinic. This was no idle threat. Steven and I had discussed the possibility many times. Living with uncertainty was wearing us both down. We wanted facts.

I evidently struck the right nerve. After that prompting, and my adding that it was abnormal for a twenty-nine-year-old woman to feel so absolutely miserable all the time, Dr. Jones sat down with me and asked me a battery of questions, some of which I thought very odd. "Are your eyes ever dry and burning?" "Is your hair falling out?" "Are you breaking out in rashes?" Then he reordered many blood and urine tests.

Two weeks later I received a phone call at work from Dr. Jones. Would I come to see him? I told him I was very tired and also quite busy. Could he not just give me all the test results over the phone? He said no, I had better come to his office.

It was a bleak December day. The long walk from my office to his wore me out. I knew something was up but still assumed it would be minor. Dr. Jones reported the various test results to me: still a low white-blood count, mild anemia, and a positive antinuclear-antibody (ANA) test. But add these findings to my aching, stiff joints; sore, weak muscles; weight loss; excessive fatigue; sore throats; breathlessness; low fevers; and sensitivity to the cold in general, but particularly in my fingers, and you are

7

in serious trouble. As Dr. Jones awkwardly said to me, "Really you have two things wrong with you. The first is not particularly serious. It's called hypoglycemia, low blood sugar. Yours is quite mild, and can easily be controlled by changing your diet, I think."

When Dr. Jones failed to proceed, and just sat at his desk staring at my file, I reminded him that he had said that there were two things wrong with me.

"Yes, uh, well, the other is not quite so simple. It's lupus. The long, medical name is *systemic lupus erythematosus* but we call it *SLE* or just *lupus*. Again, however, your case is very mild here and I don't think it's going to pose much of a problem to you. You'll be able to work and so forth. Really I think your symptoms such as fatigue and lack of energy stem more from the hypoglycemia so we'll get to work on that right away."

There were also abnormalities of my past health which, considered in retrospect, might point to lupus. I had mononucleosis at nineteen and acute anemia at twenty. After birthing Lisa at twenty-one, I promptly came down with very painful neuritis, which has been an intermittent but frequent problem for me ever since. When I was twenty-five and under a good deal of marital stress, I got shingles. Just before I separated from my husband and was caring for Lisa alone, my doctor discovered that I had less than half the number of platelets that I needed in my blood. He first took a biopsy to make sure I was at least producing platelets in my bone marrow. When it was found that I was, he put me on steroid treatment, which eventually brought the platelet level back up. If the steroids had not worked, my spleen would have been removed.

I had never heard of lupus before, but Dr. Jones managed to make one thing very clear: it was a real, honest-to-goodness *disease*, not some minor flu or infection. Although he tried hard to avoid any detailed discussion, I suppose he detected my worry and fear. He attempted to reassure me, saying that I had a mild case and that many women lead long, normal lives with lupus. Beyond that he was controlled, evasive, and quiet, fiddling with his pencil throughout our entire conversation. He obviously found it very difficult to tell me that I had a disease. To this day I believe he did not want me to understand the fullest fury that lupus could unleash on me. I am sure he thought he was sparing and protecting me. But, in reality, he was cheating me of my rights as a patient and a responsible human being. He volunteered no information about lupus and was uneasy and stilted when I shot a few questions at him. He said only that "they" did not know much about the cause, and as yet there was no cure. I should not worry, he said, just go about my normal life and "it will probably go away." I believed him, because I had always believed doctors and always obeyed them. My last question was "How serious is lupus?" to which he finally admitted, "potentially serious."

I left Dr. Jones and stumbled back to my office in the blustering cold, feeling scared, victimized, and trapped. I walked past the building in which I had met Steven years ago, yearning for him now. But he was on a business trip, and I knew that if I phoned him he would worry. Luckily everyone in my office was out to lunch, so I was able to unload and cry alone. Then I realized I could not possibly work that afternoon. Leaving a hasty note for my boss, I headed to the second-best place to Steven: my parents' house. I sobbed in my mother's arms, though I still did not fully understand what had happened to me; nor could I answer my parents' questions. All I could say was that it was an unusual, rare disease.

Now, when I look back on that day, I cannot believe my curiosity did not immediately lead me to an encyclopedia or a dictionary. I was frightened, and I clearly understood that I had an undesirable disease, even though my instincts told me that it was not mild, contrary to what Dr. Jones would have me believe. But I still made no attempt to educate myself about it. In a stupor, I only half-believed what Dr. Jones had told me, at the same time denying it, hoping he had made a mistake. Dr. Jones may not have behaved responsibly as a physician, in my estimation, because he had withheld information from me; but I did not react as a

responsible patient either. My shock and denial prevented me from
asking intelligent questions about lupus and researching it in books.

I went home to face Lisa, determined to shelter her from
distress. The show must go on as usual, I told myself. Somehow
I would break and beat this disease called lupus. Even then I did
not like the sound of the word, though I did not yet know it meant
wolf in Latin. Steven called me that night from Washington and
immediately sensed that something was wrong. Because he knew
I was due to see Dr. Jones, he put two and two together. I only
said, "I have something called lupus." Unlike me, he knew what
the disease meant. There could be no comfort for either of us
that night, only a loneliness and a foreboding gloom.

CHAPTER TWO

The Wolf Moves In

They were ... settled beasts and the possessors of a
large permanent estate with very definite
boundaries.
—Farley Mowat

Since Dr. Jones had led me to believe that my weakness and fatigue were caused by my slight hypoglycemia rather than by lupus, I began his prescribed high-protein diet. I also continued to work full-time.

Three months later my fatigue was much worse. My muscles and joints were aching continually until they reached the point where I dreaded ordinary daily activities. Folding laundry, playing the piano, typing, and mixing salads made my upper arms throb with pain. Walking long distances, standing, and climbing stairs made my upper thighs and hips ache. Often my neck was so stiff and sore that I could not turn my head without great discomfort. Dr. Jones tested my blood again and found a high lymph count. I had constant low-grade headaches, and migraines about once a week. By now, of course, it was evident that the high-protein diet had not helped. I continued it, however, because I had come to prefer protein foods, had grown accustomed to living without salt and sugar, and felt that it was basically a very healthy diet.

By the summer of 1978, after nearly a year of illness, limitations, and pain, it occurred to Steven and me that life could not continue this way. I was worse rather than better. Coping with a job and trying to be a good mother and wife at the same time was overwhelming. Furthermore, I needed even more help managing our home.

I returned to Dr. Jones and told him of my increasing problems. He did not seem to think that the sore muscles had much to do with lupus. He said I was "basically a very healthy young woman," a comment that startled me. I thought it was a very odd thing to say to a patient with a chronic disease who had come to him with numerous serious complaints. Lupus had begun to substantially interrupt my daily life. Dr. Jones said there was very little he could do for me, and suggested that perhaps I had just been working too hard lately. He advised me to take a few weeks off from work to rest, offering to write my boss a letter of explanation.

Leaning back in his chair, Dr. Jones looked at me with a smile and continued, "Yes, Joanna. That's it. A rest is what you need. Why don't you go lie in the sun for a few weeks and bake it out?"

I followed his advice, and after two weeks of potent sun I felt remarkably worse, even though I had no outward signs of lupus, like red rashes, which often occur after ultraviolet exposure. I returned to work sporting a gorgeous tan, so exhausted I could hardly think straight.

After a few more weeks passed and I failed to improve, I finally asked Dr. Jones to refer me to a lupus specialist. It was dawning on me that he did not know much about lupus or how to treat it. Reluctantly he sent me to a rheumatologist, mumbling, however, that my lupus was "mild" and "would probably go away." It was very annoying to hear those comments when my world was crumbling down on top of me. I felt threatened by my new disease, and helpless to deal with it. My ignorance of it did not help matters. It is true that at the time my case was not severe; but even low-grade lupus, or any other chronic disease for that matter, can cause drastic upheaval in a person's life, and the symptoms can be nagging and frightening.

I distinctly remember my first contact with Dr. Robert Gifford, the rheumatologist. I was lying on my bed one morning, deep into a mood of fear, when the phone rang. A cheerful voice said, "Joanna? This is Dr. Gifford. You're scheduled for a consultation with me this week and I just wanted to call you and introduce myself. I know you're probably scared. I hope very much that I can help you with your problems, and I'm looking forward to meeting you." Stunned, I did not answer him immediately. Finally I managed to thank him. When I hung up the phone I was still in shock. Did doctors really make phone calls like that? Were some of them truly that kind and sensitive? Was I dreaming? I could not believe the understanding that this man had of my situation before he had even met me. I was flattered and deeply grateful for that brief contact. Dr. Gifford accomplished exactly what he intended: I stopped worrying because suddenly I felt I would be helped, and soon.

When I finally did meet Dr. Gifford a few days later, in July 1978, he was appalled to find me so tan. He explained that exposure to ultraviolet rays can activate serious flare-ups of lupus symptoms and that for the rest of my life I would have to avoid the sun. All I could think of was Dr. Jones's recommendation that I go and "bake" in the sun. I was appalled by his ignorance. In retrospect it made me wonder whether Dr. Jones had even made my initial diagnosis without the help of other physicians.

After examining me thoroughly, Dr. Gifford sat with Steven and me for two hours in an office at the Yale–New Haven Hospital, describing lupus and all its ramifications. One thing was clear: it would *not* go away. In fact, it might get worse and more complicated; and the longer I lived the more symptoms I might have to deal with. If I were lucky I would live a long, fairly normal life, though Dr. Gifford did not agree with Dr. Jones that my case was mild. He said lupus could strike any part of my body at any time. Explaining that remission was always possible, he asserted that that would not mean the disease had disappeared permanently. Remission merely meant that the disease was "quiet," during which time I would still have to take very good care of myself. What I heard from him that morning was hard to take, but I was relieved to have the truth for a change, to be told what to do and how to handle my symptoms.

I was also very reassured to learn that most of my symptoms stemmed from lupus. That fact made it easier for me. It was comforting to think that everything emanated from a single source, and that I did not need to worry all the time about every separate problem and its origin. This realization appealed to my sense of organization. Indeed, by this time I had so many physical problems that I had begun to worry that I had more than just lupus. I could deal better with concrete facts than with uncertainty and ignorance. And I was extremely grateful to have at last found a doctor who told it to me straight. Dr. Gifford did not frighten me when he laid the cards on the table, assuming I was a responsible, capable woman who could handle my new situation. He respected my rights not only as a human being but as a patient. I was grateful for his understanding and gentleness, and I especially appreciated his honesty.

That day, though it was a sad one, marked the beginning of a close, candid doctor/patient relationship that Dr. Gifford and I still enjoy today. I was enormously relieved to have him join me in my fight. This took away some of the loneliness, and I knew that together we would make a good team in the management of lupus.

Dr. Gifford set some guidelines for me:

1. Get ten to twelve hours of sleep every night and take naps as often as needed.

2. Take twelve aspirins and five milligrams of prednisone daily for inflammation of joints and aching muscles.

3. Do not engage in strenuous sports or heavy housework.

4. Try to avoid stressful, highly emotional situations.

5. Stay out of the sun. If exposed to the sun for short periods of time, wear sunscreens and a broad-brimmed hat.

This last guideline was the most difficult of all. I was a sun worshipper and spent every spare moment each summer acquiring deep, dark tans.

It became apparent to all of us, as we discussed my symptoms, that my continuing to work full-time would be an impossibility. I no longer had the stamina required to do a good job at the office: the need for rest and relaxation was compelling. Therefore, I resigned from my job a few days later and went home to take care of myself—a task that turned out to be far more difficult than I had ever imagined. Relinquishing my job, losing contact with my working friends, threw me into an idle world where nothing awaited me but disease. I did not expect to be able to lead a happy life under such circumstances, but I was determined to give it my best shot.

I began my regimen of aspirin, prednisone, and lots of rest. As the autumn wore on, I noticed that my joints did not bother me very often any more. Once in a while my ankles or knees were stiff, and that made walking difficult; but, more often than not, it was my hips that ached from walking too much or standing too long. I got burning sensations in my legs at times. The symptoms that continued to bother me the most were fatigue and muscular soreness. And the fatigue was not the normal tiredness we all feel when we have not slept well the night before. I would wake up after twelve hours of deep sleep feeling unrefreshed, my body a lead weight. It was a fatigue that paralyzed me, left me lying motionless on my bed for hours at a time, finding it difficult to budge a muscle.

Then my muscles began to weaken. I could no longer sustain any activity for very long. The sports I had participated in—jogging, horseback riding, bicycling, and swimming—tired me easily now. I became breathless and achy after only a few minutes. My muscles also felt heavy and wooden at times. I often woke in the morning feeling as if a pile of bricks were lying on my chest. At the same time my legs were so limp—like Silly Putty—that I wondered if I could stand on them. I doubted they would actually carry me across the room. They did, but I always worried that I would fall down. This weakness was also in my upper torso. I could no longer lift anything heavy. Extending or raising my arms was extremely painful, so that simple tasks like making beds or blow-drying my hair were possible only if I was willing to endure excruciating pain.

A few months after I left my job, my mother woke up one morning, her left arm paralyzed. She had suffered a stroke and

17

had to be hospitalized. My mother's illness was extremely difficult for all of us, particularly my father. My parents had enjoyed a very close, strong marriage for over forty years. Their dreams and plans for the future during my father's retirement were suddenly shattered. I, as the only child, wanted to help him all I could with chores around his house, in spite of my physical problems. He had a housekeeper who cleaned for him, but I did his laundry, ironing, and cooked for him, certain he would otherwise starve. These tasks grew more and more difficult for me as my muscular pain increased. But my father missed his wife terribly, and I was trying to make up for his loss. I put my father first and myself last, which was undoubtedly a mistake. I outdid myself. Doing things for him that I was not even doing for my own family wore me out. Gradually I taught my father more about caring for himself, and the rest of our family chipped in too, having him for dinner several times a week and visiting my mother to give him a brief break.

What little spare energy I had this first year at home I spent on my parents and their respective problems. This added to my fatigue and tension. Because my father had no one else to turn to in emergencies, I was called to the hospital every time my mother had another stroke or crisis of any sort. Not only did I tend to my father and his needs, but I visited my mother nearly every day, as my health permitted. Although this was extremely tiring and emotionally draining—just the thirty-five minute drive in heavy traffic to her nursing home was enough to exhaust me—I *had* to see her, to bring her fresh flowers or candy or fruit, some small token of life for her to hang on to. Whatever she asked for I brought it with me the next day. What she did not think to ask for I also brought. I took care of her clothes—washed, drycleaned, and mended them, switched them seasonally, and bought whatever new things she required. I read to her, pushed her wheelchair through endless corridors, and held her hand. I stroked her head, watered her plants, hand-fed her, and occasionally brought my dogs to see her. She would rest her limp hand on their fur and feel them lick her in return, one of the few things that would raise a smile to her mouth.

I was very torn, knowing stress and exhaustion were not good for me, realizing I was not as adequate a wife and mother for all the energy and time I was pouring into my parents. On the other hand, I wanted to be involved in my mother's dying process, perhaps because of my experience with my sister. When Connie was dying of cancer in Philadelphia, I was in college in Cleveland, preoccupied with my studies, my current romance, and also recovering from mononucleosis. So when I thought about my sister, it was certainly not in terms of death. Nor did her husband or my parents choose to enlighten me. Indeed, they had told me she was in the hospital to have some cysts removed. I was later told, when I queried my parents as to why they had kept me in the dark, that, because Connie and I were so close, they and John, her husband, were afraid I would "let on" to her. I suppose they thought I would fall apart and become highly emotional with her. Then she would come to realize the severity of her condition through me. Evidently neither my parents nor John talked to her about her impending death. Because there was some small shred of hope that she might be cured by a new drug, they did not want to alarm her or me unnecessarily.

Had I been told the truth about Connie, I like to think my reaction would have been to drop what I was doing, fly to her side, comfort her, read to her, and talk with her about death. She was a highly sensitive, intelligent woman who could not possibly have spent three months in a hospital undergoing chemotherapy without suspecting that she had cancer and would die. Most likely she feigned her calm patina to soothe her family, to cause them no further worry. Being philosophical and intellectual, reading extensively, she undoubtedly spent many hours contemplating death— by herself, knowing no one else wanted to hear such talk. Why is it that people cannot talk about death? Purportedly because it brings them too close to their own mortality. But after all, death is the only concrete fact with which we live!

19

Who knows what I would have done, had I known the truth, at the age of nineteen? Nevertheless, having been deprived of taking part in my sister's death, feeling a lack of closure and an ever-present sense of unfinished business with Connie, I was determined to avoid repeating this with my mother. For now I *was* being told everything and was making crucial decisions with my father about my mother's care. I was thankful for this privilege, despite the fact that I was nervous almost every day because of it. I could not turn my back on this opportunity to help and share, lupus or not. I could not let another loved one die without me.

Meanwhile, I continued to have problems with muscular weakness and feelings of heaviness, and Dr. Gifford began to suspect the possibility of my having another disease called myasthenia gravis (MG). He also wondered if such weakness might be caused by prednisone, but since I was taking such a small amount, he doubted it. He first had to determine whether or not I was well toned and in good physical shape. I assured him I was, telling him I had always been active in sports. But we both agreed that I should go on an exercise program to see if my muscular condition would improve. I did so, even though it was difficult, considering my limited capacity for sustained activity. I tried to bike-ride every day on level ground, swam twice a week for as long as I could, and did home exercises. After a few months it was evident that exercising did not improve my muscular condition. We had established, however, that I was as toned as possible, even if I was weak and sore.

Dr. Gifford then sent me to a neurologist to get his opinion as to whether I might have early myasthenia gravis, myositis, or whether my weakness was due to lupus. After giving me many muscle tests, the neurologist concluded the last. He did find that I could not stand up on one foot from a sitting position, but apart from this he felt my weakness was unalarming. Nevertheless, he understood that it was enough to curtail many of my activities and to bring me a good deal of pain. I was relieved to know that at least he did not suspect that my muscles were deteriorating and that I did not have yet another serious chronic disease. One was more than enough.

The neurologist decided to try me on a drug called Mestinon, which is traditionally given to MG patients. He was curious to see whether this drug would help me feel stronger. I took it at noon every day, since that was when I began to tire and weaken. Mestinon did help me considerably, though it took us a while to determine how much of it my system could tolerate. When I took too much, I felt very tense and my facial muscles twitched. But, when I took the proper dose, I was less tired and did not feel the need to nap in the middle of the day. I was also able to rise on one foot from a sitting position. Because I was responding to Mestinon, there was still the lingering question in Dr. Gifford's mind whether I might have early MG. For the moment we had no choice but to accept the neurologist's opinion. I continued to take Mestinon because it was helpful, not because I had myasthenia gravis.

By this time I had voluntarily curtailed my sports. This, combined with overeating from worry and boredom, added ten pounds to my weight. Jogging had been the first to go. Gradually, when I ran, my legs came to feel so heavy I could hardly pick them up. I became very breathless and returned home to lie down. When I went riding, it got to the point where just currying and tacking a horse was exhausting work. Tired by the time I was finished, I could barely pull myself into the saddle and was not able to ride for very long. Because my leg and arm muscles had weakened, I realized I would not have much control over a horse if he got frisky. I found bicycling increasingly strenuous, too, particularly uphill. I could swim slowly for short periods, so I continued that as much as possible, along with home exercises.

This is basically the condition I was in for another year and a half. Along with the symptoms already mentioned, I periodically had nausea, loss of appetite, sore throats, and low temperatures.

Over a period of time I did manage, through dieting, to drop the excess weight I had gained. But in the winter of 1980 I got a stomach flu with excruciating lower-back pains. Valium and aspirin did nothing to alleviate the pain, so I was forced to take more potent drugs, such as Fiorinal with codeine. I tried to take as little Valium and codeine as possible, however, always conscious of avoiding drug addiction. Even after the flu left, the back trouble persisted daily and was a part of my life for more than six months.

By the spring my general health, despite the back problem, seemed to improve substantially. I felt stronger and peppier and did not tire as easily. Dr. Gifford and I decided that I should not take Mestinon any longer. I had been on it for a year, and it was debatable how much the drug was helping me. Its obvious benefits in the first few months had worn off. I also went off prednisone at this time. It was a trial—to see whether I had improved to the point where I could get along with little, if any, medication. Unfortunately, a month later my symptoms flared again. I started a low-grade fever, was extraordinarily tired, achy, and weak; and my back continued to bother me. Dr. Gifford started me on a higher dose of prednisone as well as Mestinon, hoping that both would help my strength and reduce my fever. The temperature persisted for nearly two months, during which time I had no energy at all and was in a great deal of pain from my back. Dr. Gifford increased the prednisone even more, but it still did not affect me. He was particularly surprised when this higher dose did nothing for my temperature. The flare-up continued, but just as we began to consider even larger doses of prednisone, it let up. This flare-up had lasted more than two months. When it was over, I gradually tapered back down to five milligrams of prednisone daily.

That summer I finally visited an orthopedic surgeon for my lower-back pain. He concluded that my back trouble was caused by weak muscles, which in turn were due to lupus—or at least this is how he explained it to me. There was little to do but tolerate the situation. The surgeon said that it was a chronic condition that would visit me intermittently along with my other lupus symptoms. He sent me away with a little book of exercises to follow which might strengthen my abdomen and back muscles, if indeed I were capable of strengthening any muscles at all.

Despite exercises, the back pain persisted. When, finally, I got exasperated and decided to abandon all exercising, the pain disappeared. But it was clear that I had limitations as to what my back could handle. Forget bending over to weed the garden or tie my shoes. Forget carrying heavy buckets of water to my dogs. I became cautious and learned slowly what I could and could not do without inducing the pain. When I got warning signs that I was exerting myself too much, I stopped what I was doing, rested, and gradually improved.

By this time it was late autumn of 1980. Muscular weakness and soreness continued as well as fatigue. I went through another flare-up with a low temperature for more than a month. Dr. Gifford was still suspicious of MG, so he sent me to another neurologist for a second opinion. It had become increasingly difficult for me to cut my food, drive a shift car, play the piano, type, and climb stairs, not to mention a host of other relatively simple daily tasks. This neurologist, however, like his predecessor, determined that I did not have MG or myositis. He called my muscular weakness and pain "polymyalgia" and considered it to be part and parcel of lupus. Dr. Gifford gave me a Tensilon test for MG, injecting me with a drug called edrophonium (the trade name for Tensilon). It is a quick test to see whether weak muscles suddenly get stronger. If the test is positive, it is possible that the patient might have myastenia gravis. However, my Tensilon test did not reveal any conclusive evidence.

At this time Dr. Gifford had introduced Steven and me to a rheumatologist who specialized in lupus, Dr. John Hardin. We met with Dr. Hardin several times to become acquainted with him and to hear about the lupus research he was conducting at Yale. In time Dr. Hardin became a second lupus doctor and friend to me, and his opinions regarding my condition were often helpful. He and Dr. Gifford were good friends, so they worked together easily. Because he knew prednisone had never helped me very much, Dr. Hardin suggested I try Plaquenil, often used in the treatment of malaria, but which also sometimes helped lupus patients. I started on a medium dose and, as I felt better, Dr. Gifford tapered me down to a lower dose. His overall attitude toward drugs was that the less I could get along on, the better off I would be. None of my doctors was drug-happy. But, in the spring of 1981, I came down with a virus that aggravated my lupus, and I went through another flare-up; so I returned to a medium dose of Plaquenil. I have remained on that dosage for several years. I still had some hard times, but far fewer fevers, so we all felt the Plaquenil was beneficial.

Over these few years my blood counts remained relatively the same: occasionally slight anemia, a mildly low white-blood-cell count, a high lymph count, and a positive ANA test. I continued to be very sensitive to extreme heat and cold. I had always been a summer person, but now I feared the sun, instinctively shaded myself from it, and, despite my longing for a dark tan, noticed I did not feel well in the sun. My other symptoms continued, though intermittently.

A few new symptoms became evident, however. Often my chest felt pressured, as if someone were sitting on it. Sometimes every part of my body ached simultaneously. I got sharp stabbing pains in odd parts of my body, such as my toes. Increasingly my eyes bothered me. The glands were often so dry that my eyes itched and stung. Seeing and reading were very difficult. I found myself squinting a lot, especially in the sun and under intense, fluorescent lights. I had trouble, for instance, reading the labels on canned foods in the grocery store. Dr. Gifford called this condition "Sjogren's syndrome." It was only partly relieved by "artificial tears." Being a voracious reader, I found this new symptom very annoying and depressing, as there were many days at a time when I had to strain to read a single page. I also began to have slight red rashes on my face. Sometimes they were just on my nose; other times they also fanned out onto my cheeks in the characteristic

lupus "butterfly rash." I was also beginning to experience dramatic swings in mood and energy. I was either thoroughly exhausted, my muscles heavy and stiff; or I was in overdrive, so keyed up and high-wired that I could hardly sit still. Never did I seem to be on an even keel. I was also suddenly losing my temper easily and inexplicably. When this happened at home, I could apologize to Steven and Lisa. They were forgiving, even though none of us yet understood the cause of my outbursts. My temper was far more problematic when I grew impatient and intolerant with my mother. She was pathetically sick, yet so many times I barked at her if she asked me the same question four times in a row or refused to eat or was uncooperative with her nurses. Then she would look at me with the wounded, sad eyes of a little, beaten puppy. She never said it, but I knew what was running through her mind: How can she talk to me like that when I'm so sick? As my mother's mind began to drift, she could not possibly understand what I was experiencing with my own disease. Even when I apologized, she just sat in her wheelchair and looked hurt. I carried those looks home with me, tortured with guilt and remorse.

Over the years my confidence in Dr. Jones had waned. I had therefore begun to lean heavily on Dr. Gifford. But there were times when he was out of town or busy with administrative work. We both knew I needed a good, reliable internist who knew a lot about lupus. So by the late fall of 1980 I changed to Dr. David Melchinger, whom friends, as well as my two rheumatologists, had recommended to me. Dr. Melchinger was known as a "detective" doctor who liked nothing better than to tackle a complicated case. He agreed to be my primary physician and to manage my lupus, consulting Dr. Gifford and Dr. Hardin when he felt it was necessary.

One of the first problems that Dr. Melchinger and I tackled was my mood changes and irrational flares of temper. Dr. Melchinger thought that my swings in energy and mood might be helped with the drug Lithium. My other doctors consented to a trial, though they did not hold out any great hope. I took a

low dose successfully for a week but, when the amount was increased, I had stomach cramping, severe fatigue, and my face flushed in a red rash. This larger dose, though still not very high, had given me Lithium toxicity.

We never decided how, if at all, to treat swings in energy and mood. Many times I sensed a chemical or hormonal shift occur in my body, causing me to be either depressed and tired, or pulsating with such vigor that I accomplished more in one day than others did in a week. What confused us was that sometimes, even when I was exhausted, I still felt surges of high-powered energy *within* my body, highs that made me feel very nervous and anxious, as if a jackhammer were vibrating inside me; and yet I did not have the physical power to move a limb. We were sidetracked in our attempt to deal with this symptom when another problem arose.

One day, Steven and I attended a business luncheon. I was in the midst of a flare-up and had wanted to avoid this gathering. I felt terribly shy and insecure, probably because I did not feel well enough to enter a room full of strangers and appear gracious and friendly. I had a premonition about it. When we arrived I was instinctively quiet, knowing that if I began to talk I would not make sense. Sure enough, as people asked me questions, I heard myself stammering over my words, unable to say exactly what I meant. In short, I appeared to be a dimwit, or so it seemed to me. I said very little and tried to answer monosyllabically. People probably thought I was either rude or disdainful, when all I wanted to do was leave, go home, and get into bed.

The other very frightening thing I noticed was that, when someone asked me a question, I did not fully comprehend it right away. The question did not have to be complicated either. It would take me a while to process it in my mind, sort it out, and come up with an answer, and even then, my responses were dull and made little sense. When we left, I told Steven that I would never again go into a large group of people if I felt unsure of myself.

Neither of us understood what was happening to me when these symptoms occurred.

By the autumn of 1981 these spells, as I had come to call them, occurred more and more frequently. As a result, I was increasingly frightened and began to think something was seriously wrong with my brain. I was having continuous trouble comprehending simple questions and was taking a long time to process answers. My speech was slurred, and I had to talk very slowly to get my words out precisely. Often the words that did come out were not the words I was trying to say. I felt my mind racing: so many thoughts running through it, jumping from past to present to future, that I could not concentrate on one thought at a time or remember something I had said just a minute earlier. I would dial a telephone number and then forget whom I was calling. This happened sometimes five or six times a day. I felt I had no control over my mind, over what I thought and said. My eyesight was also affected. I was extremely light-sensitive and had to wear sunglasses in a dimly lit room. Any strong light made me squint and shade my eyes. When I read, my eyes would skip randomly over a paragraph, often reading it from the bottom up, as if they could not hold to a pattern. I often read the wrong words. When I typed—and I am a fast, accurate typist—I recorded only every other word of my sentences.

Other strange symptoms appeared. Often, as I walked down a staircase, I would become disoriented, losing my sense of how many steps remained in front of me. If I failed to judge accurately, I stumbled or fell down. My facial muscles often twitched, and periodically I got tingling sensations in my arms, hands, and legs.

These spells were usually accompanied by extreme fatigue, and my whole head felt strange—as if someone were holding his hands on the sides of my head, pushing in, and squeezing as hard as he could. Because the symptoms came and went randomly, I was not suffering from them continually. They were with me often enough now, however, to be alarming.

A few particular instances drove me to discuss this new set of problems with Dr. Melchinger. One day, driving down a back road in Guilford after picking Lisa up from her piano lesson, I felt odd and suspected that I was about to have one of my spells. I was entirely disoriented and, for a quick moment, did not know where I was. Then, when I realized my location, I was not sure which side of the road I should be driving on. Nervously I asked Lisa. She looked at me with that look that children often give their parents—as if to say, "Oh, you've got to be kidding!" But then, evidently sensing my anxiety, she told me I was on the right side. I had thought I was on the right-hand side but did not know whether the right side was correct. I pulled over to the side of the road and waited for another car to come along. Then I saw I was in the proper lane after all. But I was extraordinarily unnerved and worried, even more so that Lisa had witnessed my problem when I had been trying so hard to protect her from my symptoms these past few years.

Another time, I was feeling very tired and having difficulty processing thoughts and speaking. The stereo was on. Steven asked me to turn it down. Robotically I got up and went to it. There were five knobs staring at me. Suddenly I had forgotten, after working this machine for seven years, which one controlled the volume. I looked at it, trying to figure it out. Steven finally said, "It's the one on the right." But this did not help me because I could not distinguish left from right. So I stood there until he repeated, "It's on the right, Jo." Feeling pressured to do something and not just stand there like an idiot, I turned the one on the left. When Steven impatiently corrected me, "That's the left! What's the matter with you?" I was humiliated as well as frightened.

Dr. Melchinger was impressed by what I described to him, and said it sounded like the classic kind of temporal lobe seizures that an epileptic might have. He remained very calm, reminding me that lupus can sometimes affect the brain with such seizures, reassuring me that he was certain that I did not have a tumor. Still, being the conscientious, cautious doctor he is, he ordered a brain scan and an electroencephalogram (EEG). In the meantime, despite the confidence I had in Dr. Melchinger, I was scared that I had a brain tumor. I simply could not imagine that seizures could cause the multiple cerebral problems from which I suffered. Waiting for three weeks to have my tests was agony and only gave me more time to worry. Such tests are often hard to schedule, and when I asked Dr. Melchinger to try to move them forward, he replied that he could only do so in an emergency. This response calmed me somewhat. At least my doctor did not view me as an emergency.

But many times during this waiting period I cried uncontrollably. Every person in my life took on a greater value and meant more to me than before. I clung to Steven and Lisa as never before, following them around the house like a faithful dog. And I began to wander around my home, looking longingly at each object I loved, trying to recall the stories of how and where Steven and I had acquired each, hoping I would be given enough time in my life to enjoy them all. Throughout, Dr. Melchinger was soothing and understanding. He often managed to calm me down just by a telephone call, always gently reassuring me that my problem was not going to be a tumor.

At last I had the test results. My brain scan was normal. That fact immediately dispelled my greatest fear. Unfortunately, however, I was allergic to the radiographic dye (iodine) that they injected into my system during the test. I broke out in hives all over my stomach and back, and for a few days had to take Benadryl for the itching. Still, this side effect was a minor price to pay to discover that I had no tumor. My EEG, on the other hand, was abnormal and showed "an increased cerebral excitability." This excitability was attributed to an inflammation, in my case lupus, which made me prone to psychomotor seizures.

So lupus had finally affected one of my organs—the brain. My doctors decided that my EEG, together with all the cerebral symptoms I had, pointed to central nervous system lupus (CNS lupus). I was terribly depressed, but I had lived for so many months thinking I was dying of a brain tumor that a great part of me was relieved that it was *only* this. The doctors thought that the cerebral activity might possibly account for my mood swings as well.

They hoped my seizures could be controlled with drugs and reassured me that my brain was not deteriorating. I was advised not to drive a car during my spells, that the best thing I could do for myself at such times would be to rest and not overtax my mind. The end result was that the seizures would bother me intermittently and I would have to learn to deal with them along with my other lupus symptoms.

As various diseases assaulted her over these same few years, my mother deteriorated into quadraplegia. I still did what I could for her, as far as lupus allowed. But I certainly would have done more had I not been handicapped. Before her many strokes affected her brain, she offered me her love and comfort. But beyond consolation she could not do anything for me now. Had she been well, she would have nursed me, cooked for our family, providing all those warm, wonderful functions that loving mothers perform. Once her strokes affected her reason, she could not even console me during my times of trouble. In reality I lost her long before she died. I missed her painfully, even though she remained a tremendous emotional stress for me.

Steven, Lisa, and I continued to spend as much time as possible with my father too during this time, having him to dinner several times a week, inviting him to Lisa's school plays and concerts and horse shows, even taking him on some of our vacations. What he seemed to need most was time with his family, especially time to talk to us about my mother. We were the receptacle into which he poured all his emotions about his dying wife. Although he knew very well that I had my own health problems, he was unable to deal with them beyond asking how I felt. He was totally, predictably, consumed by his wife's medical problems. His grieving had already begun. We all tried to comfort and help him, but this too took its toll on the whole family, especially on my health. There was never a moment when I was not worried about one or the other parent.

Dr. Melchinger had prescribed Dilantin for my psychomotor seizures, and all went well for the first three weeks. Then I broke out in a fine red rash all over my stomach and back, and my face was scarlet at times. Both Dr. Melchinger and a consulting dermatologist felt I was exhibiting an allergic reaction to Dilantin. Sure enough, as soon as I went off it, the rash cleared up within a few days. But this was disappointing, as Dilantin was supposedly the one drug they thought could help my seizure symptoms. During this time, to complicate matters, I came down with another virus and had to be treated with antibiotics for a few weeks. This provoked other lupus symptoms, and I felt miserable for a month. When I had recovered sufficiently, Dr. Melchinger decided, with my consent, that it would be worth trying Dilantin one more time. He said that there was a small chance that the rash I had had might have been due to lupus rather than Dilantin. It was worth it for both of us to find out, once and for all, if I could take this drug. If so, it would undoubtedly help me.

Dr. Melchinger watched my reaction as he gave me increasingly larger doses of Dilantin over a day's time. I developed a low fever but otherwise felt fine and showed no signs of a rash. Since low fevers were not unusual for me at this time, we hoped perhaps it was just a coincidence. But I went home that night, and the red rash reappeared, only this time it was all over my body and not just confined to my stomach and back. Again my face was bright red, the fever persisted, and the itching was unbearable. Clearly, Dilantin was not for me, and I resorted to Benadryl for a few days to cure the itching.

By this time I was weary of tests, drugs, allergic reactions (which I learned were very common for lupus patients), and viruses. I wanted to avoid anything but my usual, low-maintenance doses of prednisone, Plaquenil, and aspirin, and to try to get along with no new drugs. Dr. Melchinger agreed that I needed the break. Besides, my cerebral symptoms had, for the time being, subsided.

Over a period of four years, my lupus had grown from a case with no organ involvement to central nervous system lupus with minor brain involvement. We just had to hope that the seizures would not increase but would remain relatively manageable. The real problem still lay ahead—whether or not I could successfully cope with lupus on a daily basis.

The wolf, ever restless and anxious to widen his boundaries, had moved in, providing himself more territory to roam, more of my body to harass when it so suited him. Coping with lupus meant living with the wolf, whom I still regarded as the enemy. Clever at stalking his prey, now he proved adept at making himself comfortable in his newfound den.

CHAPTER THREE

The Wolf Takes Charge

The literal top dog is called the alpha male, and all
others are subservient to him. . . . An alpha animal
looks like a leader—body erect, tail held out straight or
arched high over the back, movements confident.
                                                    —Gary Turbak

After having discussed my symptoms with Dr. Gifford in our initial consultation, I was convinced that rest and the reduction of stress, neither of which I could achieve working full-time, were crucial to the management of lupus. Leaving my office and the people there who had become my close friends was one of the most difficult things I ever had to do, and was probably the most devastating blow lupus dealt me. I loved every aspect of my work — the people, the challenge and responsibility, and being part of a university environment. My job gave me purpose, identity, and self-respect. I felt needed and useful. But now, at age thirty, I was overtaken by a disease that forced me out of the mainstream, a disease that I neither wanted nor felt I deserved. I was despondent and very frightened of what lay ahead. Like a wounded animal I retreated to my lair to lick my wounds. Like it or not, a new way of life began for me.

Lisa was at camp in Maine during the time I decided to stop working, so she did not witness my most painful moments when I would cry in despair, wondering what I would now do with myself every day. By the time we visited her I had temporarily pulled myself together and was determined to spare her any worry. One day, when we were all walking through the woods at her camp, Steven dropped behind, sensing that I needed time alone with my daughter. Lisa and

I sat on a rock together looking out at Lake Sebago. She had just turned nine years old. I asked, "How would you like me to stay home with you for a change instead of working all the time?" She looked at me quizzically and asked what I meant. I could not bring myself to tell her the truth. I could not say, "Because I am sick." Instead I replied, "It occurred to me that you are growing up very fast. Before I know it, you'll be out of the house. You're my only child and I want to enjoy you. I've decided to stop working so I can spend more time with you."

Perceptively Lisa said, "But I thought you loved your job so much," to which I responded, "That's true, but I love you more." This seemed to satisfy her for the time being. She accepted it and we did not mention it further for quite a while.

I must not have been secure within myself at this time, for no sooner did I leave work than I lost all sense of identity. My confidence and determination leaked from me like a deflating balloon. The job had provided me with a title, a handy label, so I could respond with conviction when people shot those unsettling questions at me: "What do you do?" or "Do you work?" Now, instead of boldly telling them I was an administrative assistant at Yale, I recoiled, stammered, or nervously giggled. At times, I did even worse. I actually said, "I don't know," "I don't do anything," or "Nothing much." These replies immediately embarrassed me, and I became angry with myself. I knew they sounded ridiculous and only underscored my insecurity. I was aware that they humiliated Steven too, particularly when we were with his colleagues and clients. A marketing professor and an active consultant, Steven was surrounded by people who seemed highly impressed with their titles and positions. Their business talk left me cold, but it also shamed me. Now that I no longer worked, I felt I had nothing in common with them and consequently had very little to say. Stripped of my title, I was now merely "Steven's wife." I felt that people were not genuinely interested in me anymore. They perfunctorily asked what I did, then moved in on Steven, their original target. I was a mere appendage. When I had been at Woodbridge Hall, people pricked up their ears and asked me lots of questions, knowing I worked near the officers of the university, that I met celebrities through the Honorary Degrees Program—VIPs like Mikhail Baryshnikov, Leontyne Price, and Meryl Streep. That was status. They also assumed I knew big secrets about pending appointments to university posts. Now, with no job to validate me, I was inconsequential, relegated to the backburner role of faculty wife.

During the time I worked, the importance of a title had never occurred to me. Imagine telling someone that you do not know what you do! Certainly I did something. I was a wife and mother caring for her family, admittedly with help. But I did not deem this worth mentioning to engineers, bank executives, and Wall Street financiers. At that time, I would never have admitted that I had a disease and was therefore required to stay home and take care of myself. Such an admission would have seemed to be a crutch and, I was sure, they would have eyed me even more suspiciously than they already did. It would be two or three years later before I was no longer ashamed about not working. To help me regain my sense of humor and to deflect the resentment that I felt toward these high-powered workaholics nailing me to the wall and quizzing me about what I did, Steven and I drummed up all sorts of amusing responses I could supply. "I'm a taxi driver and in my spare time I do brain surgery." "I lust after tan young men." Of course I never mustered the courage to say such things. I waited until we were driving home. Then, in the car, Steven and I would privately make fun of these people, act out a possible scene, and laugh.

Rubbing shoulders with career women was especially undermining. I often found them arrogant and disdainful. Most of them turned away from me after I told them I did not do anything. I cannot say that I blame them. I am sure they assumed that I was either very stupid or very boring. Although I resented their condescension, there was a great part of me that admired them and envied them their careers. I was a modern young woman, prey to the current pressures about how women should get out in the world and be something: contribute to their families financially, use their educations, and not just sit home manufacturing babies and watching soaps. In my generation housewives were, and I believe still are, often made to feel purposeless if they stayed home tending families, insignificant if they did not have working careers, and guilty if they were not making money.

In part I shared this common disdain. I sneered at this role centered around children, PTAs, and scrubbing floors. In my first marriage, to keep myself busy as well as to add to the meager family income, I edited, typed, and proofread masters' theses and Ph.D. dissertations for local graduate students. It was not thoroughly gratifying but it beat changing diapers and watching Sesame Street. I managed this job when Lisa napped or occupied herself in her playpen. I looked upon this self-made job as a fill-in, not something I would do for the rest of my life. I dreamed that when Lisa was in school full-time I would find a satisfying career, convinced there had to be more important things to accomplish. Now, with the arrival of chronic disease, I did not want to become a housewife again. It had not yet occurred to me that there could be a middle road—that I could stay at home but still lead a meaningful life by finding something useful to do. I felt ensnared by a role I had once tested, then rejected, and now found thrust back on me. I had no choice. Circumstance, fate, call it what you will—lupus—dictated this change in my life. It was at this point that I began to hate my disease with all my energy.

Home again, I felt guilty about not carrying my own weight. I was no longer making money; in fact, a lot was now allocated toward my medical expenses. Unable to manage the household chores alone, I needed a housekeeper as well as a lot of extra help from Steven and Lisa, not to mention Kim, who did the errands and grocery shopping when I was particularly weak. The more help I needed, the more inadequate and dependent and guilty I felt. It became a cyclical, repetitive pattern.

At least I tried to make my life at home successful. I was fortunate that I had a reliable support system to begin with: a loving, patient family, a beautiful home, dedicated doctors, and my inner resources. I believe we are all born with an innate arsenal of weapons at our disposal—strength, courage, stamina, hope—and during times of crisis it is up to each of us to dig deep down inside ourselves for those tools, yank them up, and put them to good use. At the onset of my disease I was naturally preoccupied with doctors, medicines, pain, fear, and hopes for miracle cures. But over time I think I, like any patient who is sick for a long time, bucked in outrage and insult at the abuse of my body. Martialing my inner resources, I worked to improve my life. Always a fighter, I was not one to throw in the towel too quickly, no matter how many dark emotions haunted me. I was going to lick them somehow.

The first day I spent at home after resigning my job, I awakened, remembered I had nowhere to go, and cried even before I got up. After a few minutes of feeling sorry for myself, I forced myself out of bed, looking forward to nothing. I spent the day in what I would then have called an idle manner: puttering with my plants, strolling around the yard with my dog, reading a new book, and resting. But then I did make a concerted effort to prepare an excellent meal for Steven—and I hate to cook. Resenting every moment I spend in the kitchen, I often refer to myself as a "survival cook." But that day I remember telling myself that, if I could not work, then the least I could do for my husband would be to delight him with fine meals every night. I think it was a way of trying to feel worthy. We did have a gourmet spread that night, and I told Steven, "This is the first of many. You mustn't worry about me. I'll find a way to be happy at home." My excellent meals did not last long, however, because my creativity eventually led me elsewhere, primarily to writing. But whom was I deceiving that night? Steven or myself? I thought and hoped I could be content playing the happy homemaker role. Little did I realize that it was going to take much more to fulfill me.

Aside from cooking I tried to quell the ache for my old job by getting busy with projects. I delved into redecorating, needle-pointing, rug hooking, reading, playing the piano, and collecting shells on the nearby beaches, with which I made seascapes on wood. People remarked on my creativity and imagination when they saw the end results, which pleased me. But it was never enough. There was always the looming thought that I was not really good at any one thing. I was spread thin, doing many things but only halfway. What I did now, in my eyes, was unimportant. I wanted to be someone, I wanted to be recognized and appreciated for contributing something valuable to the world, but my body was holding me back. Like my wolf, all my yearnings and goals were trapped within the confines of my physicality. Nietzsche said, "He who has a why to live can bear with almost any how." For me this was an understatement.

In childhood I had been taught to be strong and proud, to put my education and talents to good use. No one prepared me for the fact that perhaps I would not be *able* to perform certain tasks. That possibility was never discussed. I entered my adult years assuming that, after I married and had children, I would make my contribution to the world in some other meaningful way. My mother was the parent who especially instilled achievement and drive in me. Her father had not allowed her to attend college, feeling that a further education was important only for men. Instead she went to Katharine Gibbs, where she trained to be a secretary. When she married my father, a college professor, she was thrown into an extremely intellectual, cultured community. Many of the other faculty wives were disdainful of my mother for her lack of education, and she suffered pangs of inadequacy and envy for years after arriving at Yale.

Fortunately, my mother was very intelligent and wanted to learn. She became a voracious reader in a wide variety of subjects. Together she and my father would spend every night after dinner reading aloud or learning foreign languages. Over time, my mother became a highly self-educated woman, greatly admired and respected by her peers, who had far more formal education than she. But she always resented her father for his shortsightedness. Consequently, she brought up her daughters to feel that education was extremely important. It was fine to marry and have children, she told us, but then there was a great deal more out there in the world, and it was up to us to take advantage of it.

And now here I was, vegetating at home all day, fooling with my meaningless little projects, tending my aches and pains—the very antithesis of my mother's and my own dreams. Interestingly enough, my mother, at the time of my diagnosis, was exceptionally understanding about my disease and limitations. She put no pressure on me whatsoever. Little did either of us know that her own illness lay only a few months away.

Rather I was the one who was hardest on myself, putting myself down for lack of achievement. Increasingly I felt restricted by the borders of my home. I missed the world of challenge and excitement. I missed people. Not a morning passed for more than a year but that I woke up and felt as if someone had thrust a dagger through my chest. I remembered I did not have to work. I did not have to go anywhere. No one was waiting for me. No one wanted me.

In the meantime, Lisa's awareness of my condition was gradually increasing. She no longer believed I had stopped working just to be with her. An observant, alert child, she began to notice my various symptoms, particularly the fatigue and arthritis. But by far the most obvious signal to Lisa that something was wrong with her mother was that I had to curtail some of my activities with her, primarily riding. She also noticed that I often asked her to help me with chores I had previously done myself but which now caused me great pain, simple tasks like ironing and sweeping. Gradually Lisa began to question me: "Why can't you ride with me anymore?" "Why are you always so tired?" "Why does it hurt you to walk up the stairs?" "Why do you stay out of the sun now? You always loved the sun."

I finally had to sit down and have a long talk with Lisa. This was very hard for me because it came at a time when I was desperately trying to deny my disease and to hide it from the world. I did not enjoy discussing it. Least of all did I want to talk about it with my daughter. My maternal instinct was to protect her from this unwelcome intruder as long and as much as I possibly could. But confrontation was inevitable.

Our first conversation was short and simple. I gave Lisa the bare facts about lupus, just enough information to satisfy her curiosity but not so much as to frighten her. I told her as much as I felt a child of ten could understand and digest.

I reassured her, "Yes, it's a disease which sometimes brings me pain. But I'm very fortunate that I can live at home here with you and Daddy. As long as I rest a lot and take my medicine I'm going to be fine. It's just that there are now some things that I can't do with you anymore."

"Yeah, like riding. I really miss that. We always went riding together. Isn't there any way you can ride again?"

"I don't think so, Lisa, not unless my muscles get a lot stronger. You wouldn't want me falling off and hurting myself more, would you?"

Hanging her head, Lisa said, "No, of course not." After a short pause, she then asked, "Am I going to get lupus too?"

There it was. Lisa had listened attentively, then zeroed in on the question I had dreaded the most. Shrewd child, I thought, as I emphatically replied "No." I did not yet suspect that lupus could be passed on from parent to child, so I was not lying. I truly did not think Lisa could inherit it from me.

Next she asked, "Are you going to die?"

Oh boy. Another big one. Pulling myself together, I said, "Just like everybody else I'm surely going to die someday. But not until I see you grow up and get a job and find a nice husband and have babies and make me an old grandmother!"

She laughed. Again I reassured her that I would live a long life if I took good care of myself.

Lisa seemed to believe me and handled the whole conversation in a very mature manner. She did not appear to be overly concerned or anxious about lupus or me. I think she was grateful to understand at last why I could not keep up with her anymore and why I needed so much extra help. She became very considerate of me once she understood my condition, often reminding me not to lift heavy grocery bags, taking me by the arm to help me up a staircase, or rubbing my back and legs when they hurt. To this day she is still the best backrubber I know!

On the other hand, the two "big" questions had in fact already occurred to Lisa, which surprised me. If she had been worrying about the possibility of inheriting lupus or about my death, she had not let on. Years later she admitted she indeed had been very frightened that I would die while she was still a child. I do not believe she worried about this longer than a few months, but it was nevertheless of primary concern to her for a while. She relaxed about it only as time passed and as she witnessed my ability to manage the disease at home.

I always hoped Lisa was still too young for my condition to make a real impact on her. Most important, I did not want her to remember me as an invalid during her childhood years. She was already being exposed to enough sickness, watching her grand-mother die slowly before her eyes. So, even when I was not feel-ing well, I tried to be up and dressed, and I kept my requests of her to a minimum. I leaned far more heavily on Steven, feeling that he, as an adult, could handle it better.

But at the same time that I tried to hide my symptoms, Lisa often overheard conversations with either Steven or my doctors when I talked with them on the phone about my problems. I went out of my way to closet myself in a private room but, being the curious child she was, nine times out of ten I could count on her barging in. Gradually I stopped being so afraid of discussing lupus in her presence. I relaxed because she seemed to take it in stride. Sometimes she would ask me a question about lupus and catch me off guard; but in time I was able to give her a straight answer, cautious not to scare her but trying to be honest. If the two "big" questions still bothered her, she was a great actress.

Lisa was nearing eleven at this time and relied on me less and less as she grew more independent. Certainly she needed me in her own way, but not to manage her life completely the way a mother does for a very young child. Now she no sooner popped in the door to say hello after school than she was off and running around the neighborhood with her friends. I felt dismissed and superfluous. Why did I need to be there? Merely to open the door for her at three in the afternoon? In case she fell off her bicycle and required a Band-Aid? Of the two of us, I was by far the needier.

Steven had begun to travel more. He was often out of town with clients or attending conferences, so I did not feel particularly needed by him either. In fact, his travels only widened the increasing gap between us. Before the onset of lupus, there were few activities that Steven and I engaged in without each other. Sports as well as cultural events played an important role in our lives together. We believed that marriage should be nurtured by sharing ideas and values as well as activities to the greatest extent possible. Although I could still go to a play or a concert, I was forced to abandon sports, which abruptly removed me from a great part of my family's life. The sting was deep.

I was miserable every time one or both of them left without me. Of course I realized that, just because I could no longer participate in these activities, it did not mean that my family should have to give them up as well. Even when I felt very alone and left out I *tried*, often unsuccessfully at first, to allow Steven and Lisa their pleasures in life without resentment, reminding myself not to manipulate them with guilt just because they were healthy and I was sick, because they were free and I was restricted. I knew that they had problems of their own directly related to my disease. The least I could do was try to spare them my feelings of jealousy and hurt, to encourage them to carry on as normally as possible, sometimes with me, but more often without me. Suddenly I was required to watch them do the doing. I was on the outside of their lives now, yet I desperately wanted to be with them, sharing.

The most distinct memory I have of the distance growing between Steven and me was when we went to Antigua for a week alone together. It was our first vacation without Lisa in a long time and, unbeknownst to Steven, I looked upon it romantically, as a second honeymoon. Steven, on the other hand, had clearly come to Antigua for fun and sports, sun and people. Neither of us had anticipated how much the hot, sunny climate of a Caribbean island would divide us. It was the worst possible choice, for me at least. As it turned out, we might as well have taken separate vacations.

Upon our arrival at Galley Bay a young native named Eugene, who worked as a cabin boy, carried our bags to our thatched-roof hut. The first question Steven asked him was, "Are there any good places around here to run?" Eugene told him about the beautiful mountain paths along the sea. Steven next asked if he would like to join him, and they set a time for six o'clock the following morning. There it was: within ten minutes of our arrival I was already feeling left out and replaced. Steven, intent upon pursuing his interest, as well he should have, merely found himself a new partner, knowing I could not jog with him. That it seemed to come so easily to him was the wound that smarted the most. Still I reminded myself not to be a killjoy, to be a good sport and let at least one of us have some fun.

Unfortunately, my back problems kicked up in Antigua and I spent a good part of the week lying flat, getting by on piña coladas or Valium to quell the pain. When I felt well I wandered the beaches, collecting shells, or sat in the shade reading, watching Steven bake in the sun. Before the week was out, Steven had jogged every day with Eugene, sailed, and snorkled. This last activity intrigued him. He often left to investigate the coves and inlets with his newfound friends.

Although the weather was fickle and the cockroaches multitudinous, we did have some fun together too, despite my intermittent back pain. But, regardless of what we did as a couple, I always felt like Steven's leftover, the person he turned to at the end of the day once he had finished his frenetic sports agenda. Excluded on many counts, I longed for his companionship in a way he could never possibly have imagined.

Steven was not deliberately insensitive. A rational man, he was just going about the business of life, figuring that, if I could not accompany him in his ventures, he would either do them alone or find new partners. It was that simple. His restless nature and his apparent need to release vast sources of energy compelled him to work hard and play hard. As far as he was concerned, I, left to my own devices, was shaping my new life successfully. I doubt it ever occurred to him that I felt so excluded and miserable. Little did he know and little did I say, a big mistake that only underscored our growing lack of communication. Deep down the possibility had also occurred to me that Steven was deliberately spending a lot of time away from me, not only because I was unable to join him in his pursuits but also because I was no longer good company. This needled me so much that I tried, unsuccessfully, to repress it.

I never revealed my feelings to Steven. I just bit my lip and tried to fake a nonexistent joie de vivre. I endeavored to appear unselfish and enthusiastic whenever he did something without me. If there is anything I loathe it is a whiner, so I tried not to complain. I knew, *rationally,* there was no reason why Steven should not continue his activities, whether I could be with him or not. *Emotionally,* however, the situation was unacceptable to me. But I have never been a good faker. More often than not, stifling my true feelings simply made me short-tempered and moody. If Steven tried to find out what I was unhappy about, I declined to explain. I knew this was unfair, but I was not yet at a point where I could articulate my feelings. I was struggling to accept them and kept hoping that I would, in the end, succeed.

I often thought during this time that, had I been married to a different type of man, a quiet, introverted sort, for instance, perhaps I would not have felt such a contrast between us. It was because Steven was successful and energetic that he unwittingly emphasized my inabilities. He was vivacious, dynamic, independent—an achiever always. I was sluggish, static, dependent—an achiever only when my health permitted. More and more I feared I would not be able to keep up with him enough to hold his interest. I sensed that he needed and deserved a healthy wife who could participate in his activities, be his companion as I once had been and now could be only in limited respects. It never occurred to me to look around at other marriages. Had I done so I would have realized that in almost no marriage are the mates constantly together; nor do they always choose the same interests. Often one likes tennis and the other sings in a choir. Or one is an avid jogger and the other a gourmet cook. Everyone needs some personal space, some time alone to himself. No one wants to be choked and restrained by a relationship. We need to encourage one another to grow, and if we undertake a separate activity now and then it does not necessarily mean that we do not love each other or that we cannot enjoy a strong partnership. Much later I learned the value of Steven's continuing to pursue his own life. He would inevitably have built up a resentment toward me had I demanded that he give everything up and "be sick" along with me. But my marriage was young—only six years at this point— and it was my second. I was determined to preserve it, so I clung to Steven like a parasite, as daily I felt chronic disease testing and threatening us and our marriage.

I began to resent Steven for the very fact that he was working, that he got up every morning and left the house eagerly, returning refreshed and stimulated by his teaching and consulting. Again, logic told me he had to work, to fulfill himself as well as to take care of the family. Certainly he was not expected to stop working now, especially when I was sick. But his work also brought him a great deal of satisfaction and pride. It was this I held against him, probably because my own pride was nonexistent. I desperately needed to point to something in my own life that gave me self-respect and dignity. I searched and found nothing.

Unfortunately, my resentment of Steven led me to withdraw from him. Finding it very difficult to relate to him when he came home from the office, I did not want to hear about anything he had done during the day. This was a big change for him. Steven was accustomed to sharing everything with me. He would invariably burst through the door at six and begin telling me the high points of his day. I listened to him in silence, busying myself around the kitchen, trying to let it all pass through me, numb. But my bitterness grew like a cancer within me. I harbored it and allowed it to fester into a hatred toward the one person with whom I wanted to share my life. I kept quiet about my feelings, still expecting them to magically change into acceptance. But week after week, month after month dragged on, and I cried when Steven left for work. I finally taught myself to sleep later in the morning, so late that when I woke up he was gone. Then I did not have to face kissing him goodbye and trying to be cheerful when I said, "Have a good day." And all afternoon I braced myself for his return when I knew that he, in his usual, talkative, open manner, would relay every move he had made, every meeting he had attended, what every faculty member or client had said. Steven was either impervious to my silence or he had decided to ignore it.

What I was really angry about was lupus and the difficult changes it brought to my life. I was not angry with Steven nor did I hate him. I hated lupus and the limitations it imposed upon me. My hatred of it made me envy and resent *all* people who were healthy and who worked or who participated in activities that brought them satisfaction. Ironically, I felt most content and self-assured with housewives, who posed no threat to me, for I did not have to defend myself to them.

Worst of all I hated myself. Undoubtedly this was the well from which my anger and envy of others flowed. I could not look at myself and be proud. This brewed constant discontent inside me. I retreated into books and music, often blasting my feelings out on the piano, pounding the keys as hard as I could with melancholy tunes. It became my refuge. Better to abuse the piano, I thought, than Steven or Lisa. It is a truism that those who are unhappy with themselves lack the ability to be happy about anything else. The entire world looked dim to me. I joined the ranks of the malcontents.

Self-hatred bred self-pity. This frightened me because it was so contrary to the way I had been brought up. The virtues of self-control and inner resilience had been drummed into me since I was a little girl. My mother, a strict, stoic New Englander who placed a very high priority on self-reliance and privacy, brought me up with many maxims which still keep me on track today: "If you can't do something right then don't do it at all." "If you can't say something kind then don't say anything." Her most important was "Don't wear your heart on your sleeve." She meant that I should not complain during times of adversity, that I should be especially careful never to burden others with my problems. Everyone, she reminded me, had problems, and the last thing they wanted to do was listen to mine. Instead I should face them directly and try to resolve them by myself. It was unacceptable to whine and moan. If ever I complained or felt sorry for myself, I could count on no attention from my mother.

During my childhood I spent many happy summers at Singing Eagle Lodge on Squam Lake in the White Mountains of New Hampshire. My camp director, Doc Ann (Dr. Ann Gibson), hailed the same virtues my parents were trying to instill in their daughters. Doc Ann reminded me of my resilient maternal grandmother, a woman who lived courage and determination every day of her life. When her husband lost his job and most of his assets in the crash of 1929, they were forced to remortgage their house and take out loans on insurance policies. My grandfather lapsed into a depression. It was Hannie who held the family together. Against her husband's wishes she took a job at a nearby Electrolux factory to help make ends meet. This must have been a difficult adjustment for a well-bred lady of society, the wife of a formerly successful New York businessman who once owned a thriving advertising agency. With never a complaint she relied on an inner core of steely strength, while outwardly managing to remain warm and loving.

The models of my mother, Doc Ann, and Hannie were always before me, inspiring me to be strong, nagging at me when I was weak. In contrast to these examples, I knew, during my first

49

difficult years of lupus, that negative emotions were controlling me, molding me into an ugly person. I had not yet learned to turn these feelings into something that worked *for* me rather than against me. So I not only despised myself for not doing something worthwhile, my own behavior disgusted me. I was my own worst enemy.

Because of my self-pity, anger, and hatred, I grew increasingly contrary and reclusive, refusing to talk to Steven about much except essentials. I told him, "I'll talk when I'm ready. I don't know yet what's bothering me. I can't say it in words." What I really wanted to say was, "I hate you. I hate the world. I hate everyone who is healthy and going to work every day. I hate being left out." All the while, these exhausting, unattractive emotions warred inside me, tangled themselves up in each other until I could no longer separate them and deal with them. They screamed at me all day long until my head spun. I had no inner peace.

I turned into a shrew. Fighting back the only way I knew how, I took pot shots at the one person I needed most. For every success Steven brought home, I made snide remarks. I even found myself making derogatory comments about him in mixed company. Of course, it did not make me feel better when I criticized him, only ashamed when I heard what I was saying. I embarrassed Steven as well as our friends, yet I continued. I had some morbid need to get revenge, to punish this healthy man. Subconsciously I must have felt that, if I undermined his successes, my own failures would not be so glaringly apparent. Perhaps, if I raked him over the coals long enough, I could bring him down to my level, where he would be more human, less perfect. Certainly I was very proud of Steven, but I could not admit it to myself or others. Every ounce of pride I invested in him was pride I did not have in myself.

Once in a while my ill temper could be attributed to psychomotor seizures. But more often than not I was just plain angry that I was sick and everyone around me was well. I was also irritable with Lisa. But I made a far greater effort to control my emotions around her, keeping in mind that she was just a child and would not understand the source of my anger and frustration as Steven would. When I did lose my temper with her I always apologized later, explaining that it was because I had been tired and achy, not because she had done anything to provoke me. She was usually understanding, forgiving, and, I believe, pleased to see that a parent was capable of making an apology.

During these first years at home I channeled what little energy I had into destructive, gloomy emotions. Although they dominated me, I knew I was aiming them at the wrong targets. Lisa was maturing beautifully and Steven was not doing anything different from what he had always done. He remained a devoted, loving husband and father. He worked hard, not only for his own sense of achievement, but also because he was a dedicated family man, intent on supporting Lisa and me to the best of his ability. He had not changed. I had—and so drastically that I did not even recognize myself. Having a good time, with my family or anyone else, was such a rarity that I forgot how to laugh—at life as well as at myself. When you lose your sense of humor, you know you are in troubled waters.

No longer was I in control of myself, emotionally or psychologically. I had allowed the wolf to take charge. Deftly he had clawed his way to the depths of my soul, where he perniciously chewed on my optimism, my sense of self-determination, and my usual generosity toward others. Once he had moved in, I had at least hoped to leash him. Now I was the one trapped, collared, straining for freedom.

CHAPTER FOUR

The Wolf Marks His Territory

I am sure that my anger and hatred toward others and myself stemmed directly from my denial of lupus. I did not yet accept it as part of my life. It embarrassed and shamed me. I had great difficulty admitting that I had a disease, especially such an odd one as lupus. People wondered why I left my job so suddenly. At first they assumed I was pregnant. But when, months later, I showed no signs, they pressed me to find out why I had retreated back home. I feared telling them, knowing they would say, "Lupus? Never heard of it. What's that?" and then I would have to explain. But it was not only my dread of explanation that prevented me from telling people I had lupus. I hated the very sound of the word, and its meaning even more. When I said "Lupus," I felt strange and self-conscious. It was not like saying "I have mononucleosis" or "I have a cyst on my ovary." Lupus sounded like some sort of alien fungus to me and always required definition. I feared that people might even suspect I had invented the word, it sounded so far-fetched. I did not want them to find out that it meant "wolf." Perhaps they might think it was contagious and avoid contact with me.

More than a year passed before I began, tentatively at first, to tell my secret; and even then I was very selective about my audience, choosing close friends whom I knew would be gentle and understanding. But, even when I mustered the courage to speak up, I found myself saying "I have an illness" or "I have a disease," rather than "I have lupus." It was a long time before that word came easily to me, before it slid off my tongue without my heart pounding. The poet Maxine Kumin once said, "Naming things is a way of owning them." This was my very problem: if I named lupus I would be admitting it, incorporating it into my life, owning it. I was still unprepared to do this.

In sum, this bizarre disease made me feel tainted, stigmatized. I would never be the same woman again. The odd nature of lupus made me feel strange. Consequently, I felt removed from others— different, weird, a kind of freak. This was a very cyclical problem, for the odder I felt, the less inclined I was to talk to others about lupus. It then became even more unlikely that I would admit the disease to myself.

My feelings of inadequacy prevailed. My outward appearance remained fairly normal, but I was painfully embarrassed by arthritis, even though it was intermittent and infrequent. I did not want people, particularly Steven, to see me hobble down the street because of aching hips or slowly drag myself up a staircase because of sore muscles. I was in anguish whenever Steven had to cut my food when we dined out, especially if we were with other people. Such limitations made me acutely self-conscious, and slowly I began to see myself as an unattractive woman. How could I be otherwise when I was stained and disabled by a disease? How could I play the part of an energetic, bright, attractive woman when my illness continually held me back and weighed me down? Because I felt ugly and afflicted within myself, I assumed I must appear that way to the rest of the world. No matter how many compliments Steven paid me, nor how much attention he showered upon me, I still thought I had let him down. I was no longer the woman he had married. His cheerful, positive, spunky partner had vanished. Her replacement was irritable, negative, sluggish, and extremely hard to live with.

To counteract such feelings of inadequacy I made a strong effort to look good, even when I was sick. At first I got out of my jeans and sweatshirts and began to wear office clothes again. But that phase did not last long because it was impractical. Steven came home from work and changed out of his suits into old corduroys. He looked at me and asked how could I possibly spend my days walking the dogs or gardening in dress clothes. So I resorted to wearing jeans again—my natural look, and really the way Steven preferred me—but I still made sure they were neat and clean, and I wore them with sharp sweaters and jackets. Because Steven worked with interesting, stimulating women every day, I had to look my best for him. It is unfortunate that at this time in my life I dressed well solely for the sake of my husband. Personally I could not have cared less what I wore. I did not like my self, much less my body. I was so bored and unhappy that what I put on made no difference to me. However, I knew Steven appreciated my efforts.

I would be less than honest if I ignored one of the most important ways a woman is a wife to her husband—sexually. My feelings of imperfection and unattractiveness increased, naturally, when lupus flared and left me exhausted, stiff, and sore. During those times, I literally could not raise my arms to embrace Steven. Every limb was so weak and leaden, I could not respond sexually, nor, obviously, did I *feel* sexy. Abstinence was certainly not the solution, however. When my condition lasted for a long time, sometimes months, I was acutely aware of being an inactive participant. But the closeness comforted both of us. This was when I needed Steven to be especially loving and undemanding, because I felt all the more inadequate and frustrated. He never once failed me.

Of all my emotions, fear was the most prevalent. Even though I had yet to research lupus, I at least knew it could be very serious, that it could kill, even if rarely. Consumed with the idea of dying young, I often woke in the middle of the night, thinking in horror that I might die soon, that I might not be able to watch Lisa grow up, that Steven might replace me with another wife. Those nights I could not fall asleep again. The longer I lay there worrying the more frightened I became, my thoughts growing gloomier and, as is usual during the night, out of perspective. Feeling completely alone, I was often tempted to wake Steven for comfort, but I never did. I just lay closer to him, consoled by his presence and physical warmth, thinking that he had a full day ahead and certainly did not need me to deprive him of sleep. Because I was able to live at home with my chronic disease and had not yet seen the inside of a hospital room (not for lupus anyway), perhaps I had no rational cause to think about death. Nevertheless, the fear persistently gnawed the back of my mind. Just knowing the *potential* of lupus was enough to frighten me. Having to watch my mother's agonizingly slow dying process only added to my fears about my own death.

Steven often tried to calm me with the argument that people are run over by cars unexpectedly or have sudden heart attacks without any previous history of illness. In other words, people can die anytime. No one is told when, where, or how. We all begin to die from the time of birth. I was not special simply because I had a disease. But these thoughts did not pacify me. I was scared of the unknown. What lay ahead? How much pain might there be? Would I live only a few more years, or would I be blessed and live to be an old grandmother as I had promised Lisa? Now that my brain was slightly affected by lupus, would the illness move to my kidneys next, requiring dialysis?

By far the most unsettling fear was that I might have transmitted my disease to my daughter. This thought had not occurred to me right away because Dr. Jones had distinctly told me that lupus was non-hereditary. It was only when I began to reread Flannery O'Connor that this fear overwhelmed me. Although I knew O'Connor had died of lupus, I had not realized that her father also had had lupus. This was when I first discovered that the disease *could* be passed from parent to child. My doctors reassured me that Lisa's chances of contracting lupus were minimal, one in a hundred or more, that statistics showed that only rarely was lupus inherited. Still, I now knew it was a *possibility*, and at this time in my life, when I felt everything else was against me, I had little reason to sustain any hope that Lisa would be spared.

Once this fear seized me, it persisted. Only time, over a period of four to five years, wore it down. Time, constantly reading the statistics in medical journals, and listening to my ever-comforting doctors: "To worry about Lisa getting your disease is a waste of time. You cannot predict her future. If she does get it, there's nothing you can do about it. Just remember the facts are on your side."

No matter what anyone did, nothing could change the fact that I was a mother and my child was a part of me. She had lived inside my body, had come from my body, after all; my body was therefore now in hers. Now she was carrying me. I was miserable every time I thought about it. I used to tell Steven, "If Lisa gets this damn thing I'll never be able to live with myself. I would feel responsible. I already feel guilty and nothing's happened." Steven rationally tried to calm me, but my fear overpowered reason.

I was also afraid of prolonged hospitalization or further organ involvement. The possibility of lengthy steroid treatment frightened me because it would cause multiple damages to my body as well as inflate it like a balloon. As the lupus progressed, I also came to fear the seizures because they signified a loss of control over my body, particularly my mind.

I was also concerned about being dull and uninteresting to my husband. Would he return home at the end of the day and find me boring? I no longer had much to say to him. After his exciting report of his day's activities, mine paled in comparison. I could say only that I had done the laundry, driven Lisa to her piano lesson, fed the dogs, or some other mundane activity. None of it sufficed. I felt unworthy. How could a man sustain an interest in a woman who did not do or say anything scintillating? If I did talk, it usually concerned lupus—my various doctor visits, exams, drugs, lab tests, their results, and so on. After a while I felt self-conscious and hypochondriacal. I was suddenly an invalid.

Consider the meaning of the word. I was *invalid*. Steven was now my caretaker. I resented the role change. Previously, we had fashioned a marriage of equality. Now everything was turned upside down and I was deprived of my equal status. Slowly I was becoming a financial and emotional drain on my husband. Burdening him was bad enough, but would I be able to *keep* him? I was consumed with fear of losing him even though he had never given me any cause.

Then a new fear entered the scene. After my mother had been ill for quite a while, a doctor who was new on her case stopped me in the hallway of the hospital one day and said, "I understand you have lupus. I'm interested in following up on that. Your mother clearly has a vascular disease among her many other problems, and since lupus can sometimes affect the vascular system, there may be a correlation here." I was aware that lupus was a connective-tissue disease; what I had not realized until then was that lupus could also affect the vascular system. Stunned and panicked, in one lightning second, standing there in that cold, antiseptic hospital corridor with some strange man I had never seen before, it occurred to me that possibly my mother had transmitted lupus to me.

I asked my mother's personal physician to test her for lupus. Indeed, her antinuclear-antibody test was just slightly positive and of only questionable significance. Her strokes were characteristic of large-vessel thrombosis, unusual for lupus, and she had never exhibited any other manifestations of lupus, so lupus was not diagnosed. Her doctor stressed the fact that many people can have positive ANA tests and never get lupus. Indeed they can register positive ANA tests and have entirely different diseases. He said the relationship between our physical problems was cloudy and would be difficult, if not impossible, ever to determine.

I do not remember the name of the doctor who questioned me about lupus that day in the hospital, but I wish I had never met him. He was doing the normal detective work that a good physician must do to investigate and solve a complicated medical case. But he also succeeded in terrifying me, and it took a lot of time and reassurance from other doctors before I believed I had not inherited lupus from my mother, at least not directly. It was a puzzle that no one ever fitted together. I forced myself to think that my mother did not have my disease, and I hoped and prayed every day of my life that Lisa would not get it either. A smoldering fear remained. I may have managed to convince myself that my mother did not have my disease, but I was sure there was *some* connection between our two cases. Furthermore, now that I realized that lupus could touch the vascular system, I began to have nightmares about having strokes. I suppose that again this was natural, considering that I was a first-hand witness to the severe damage that a series of strokes had done to my mother. For several years I tried to learn to live with these various fears, hiding them deep within myself. But they often got the better of me, and I would break down and call either one of my doctors or a close friend for comfort. I did not turn so often to Steven, not wanting to overload his capacity for sympathy and support. He was already doing so much for me. I assumed he must have a breaking point, that there was only so much of me and my chronic disease that he could take. So I tried to spare him as much as possible, as I did Lisa, knowing they must be scared too, though they never mentioned it.

Loneliness was another difficulty, because it was always with me, like the fear. My working friends had little extra time for me, and as yet I had not met new people in Guilford. A natural loner, preferring to be with others on my own terms, I had not tried to meet anyone or pursue any new interest that would enable me to make friends. I remained solitary and reclusive, relying solely on my family for friendship. I was especially lonely when lupus was exacerbated and I was confined to bed for weeks or months at a stretch. But, after living through many flare-ups, I came to realize that I was indeed alone with my disease. No matter how many people loved, supported, and comforted me, no matter how many doctors were working hard for me, it was ultimately up to me and me alone to deal with the illness mentally and physically. No one else could take on the aches and pains, or the loneliness and fears, and manage them for me. I was the patient who must learn patience. I was the warrior with, as yet, no army.

The isolation was real and cold. While it is true that many other people have lupus, or other chronic diseases, even they can do little but empathize. I, with my own particular symptoms, therapy, and emotional problems, was called upon to rally, to rise above lupus and conquer it each time it flared. The expectation was overwhelming, the loneliness devastating. Flannery O'Connor once wrote in a letter to a friend, "In a sense sickness is a place, more instructive than a long trip to Europe, and it's always a place where there's no company, where nobody can follow." How insightful, savage, and true.

Under normal circumstances, I would have turned to my mother for support. If anything was appealing about staying home, it was more companionship with my family. My mother had played a key role in my life. We shared many common interests and thoroughly enjoyed one another's company as we traipsed through art galleries, antique stores, or took long walks on the beach. I relied on her for comfort and advice. She was a great source of intellectual stimulation too as she constantly fed me books to read. We had experienced only a few hard times during our mother/ daughter relationship, misunderstandings which, in the long run, proved to strengthen the bond between us. But now she was losing the battle of life just when I needed her the most. This only served to add to my sense of loneliness. With my sister dead, my mother dying, and my father completely preoccupied with my mother, I felt orphaned. Yes, I had Steven and Lisa. But my family of origin, the family with whom I had grown up and on whom I would normally rely for comfort and support, had vanished.

While I watched my mother deteriorate and fought my emotions concerning lupus, I was often dealing with the random and various physical symptoms of the disease. One day I would feel fine, sprinting around the house with childlike energy, and the next day I was down with a one-hundred-degree temperature, aching joints, and exhaustion, which was often accompanied by my cerebral symptoms. This would last anywhere from one day to three or four months. Sometimes my ankles hurt so much I could not walk. Another day I had sharp, stabbing pains in my shoulders. I felt like a chameleon, or worse, a hypochondriac, for every time Steven asked me what was wrong and where I hurt, I had something new to report. The disease crept all over me, traveled through my body, affecting me literally from head to toe. I did not understand what was happening to me, but I knew I had lost control over my body. Before lupus, if I was overtired, a nap was a speedy remedy. Now the fatigue persisted, despite naps and long sleeps at night. Before lupus, if I had a fever and sore throat, it was usually labeled "a cold." I went to bed for a few days and it disappeared. Now these symptoms stayed with me for months at a time.

It was also difficult to continually visit doctors, undergo examinations, try out new drugs, and the like. I trusted all my doctors, but they were often frustrated by my condition and sometimes were at a loss as to what to do with me. Their bewilderment made me apprehensive and filled me with premonitions. When, however, they succeeded in coming to some concrete resolution, some clear way to handle a particular symptom, I was better able to cope. Due to my sense of organization, I found it far easier dealing with a specific problem than dwelling in limbo where I was a medical enigma. One of my doctors once referred to me as "a celeb[rity] around town," because at that point about four different physicians were trying to figure me out. This made me feel special, in a good way, but it also frightened me. So, though I liked my doctors and had faith that they were working hard to help me, I often dreaded my visits to them for fear of learning bad news or witnessing their frustration.

But it was not the actual physical aches and pains I found so difficult to endure. As they became a part of me, I gradually grew accustomed to them. I learned to sustain periodic discomfort with the aid of various drugs as well as a blossoming facility to ignore such unpleasant aspects of my life. I also discovered that it is possible to train oneself to live with pain, because in time its severity lessens, or at least I perceived that it did. Mounting a staircase with sore hips did not hurt so much on the seventh day as it did on the first. If folding sheets continually shot burning pain through my shoulders, I did at last get used to it. The pain was still there, of course. It had merely become a "normal" part of my life to which I had accommodated myself.

Rather, it was more the unpredictability and uncertainty of lupus that I found exasperating and hard to live with. The attacks came with no warning, no regularity, no apparent reason. I never knew what to expect next. Powerless, I was victim to a disease that invaded and possessed my body, then whimsically toyed with it—the wolf playing with his prey, first hunting it down, then tearing it to pieces, resting awhile as the victim lies before him slowly bleeding, then at last moving in for his final feast. And I was frustrated by the hit-and-run nature of lupus. I wanted to drag my wolf out into the open and wrestle with him until one or the other of us became the established leader. I had been used to peace and order in my life. Now this intruder came and went, did its dirty work on my body, then vanished, only to reappear suddenly, never when it suited me or fitted neatly into my life. Indeed, it seemed that lupus surfaced at precisely the most inconvenient times, making long-range planning impossible, and even daily planning difficult.

At the end of a long flare-up I would emerge slowly, skeptically, feeling drained but relieved as the shroud lifted. It took at least a month until I could feel that perhaps my strength was restored forever. But I learned, after many many disappointments, that lupus would resurface to take over again and devour my energy.

A cyclical pattern arose. Pain and inconvenience aside, the variety and randomness of the symptoms often induced the very emotions I was trying so desperately to control. It seemed that every time I began to get a handle on fear and self-pity, another flare-up would slap me down and, once again, the physical problems triggered the emotional ones. This often led to severe depression. If depression is anger turned inward, I was easy prey. Days passed when I lived in a stupor, feeling sorry for myself, hating my life, imagining the worst, dreading the future.

When the symptoms began to subside, my inner self began to lighten. After experiencing this pattern many times, I thought that, if the mind were so dependent on the body, I could perhaps reverse the pattern and make the body dependent on the mind. If my physical condition could so negatively affect my mind, perhaps my attitude and spirit could positively affect my body, thereby lightening the impact of flare-ups. At least I had some control over my mind. Dr. Viktor E. Frankl, the famed psychiatrist who founded logotherapy and who survived three years in Nazi prison camps, wrote in his book *Man's Search for Meaning,* "Everything can be taken from a man but one thing: the last of the human freedoms— to choose one's attitude in any given set of circumstances...." Certainly I had not chosen lupus, it had chosen me. But now a different sort of choice presented itself to me. I could at least choose my *attitude* toward my chronic disease.

Experimenting, I noticed that, when I succumbed to depression, I felt worse. But, when I occasionally managed to boost my spirits and think positively, the symptoms did not seem so threatening and the world and my future looked brighter. One flare-up after another demonstrated to me the absolute necessity of my body and mind working together in combination, as a team, since they were evidently so highly dependent upon one another. However, this is easier said than done, and I do not mean to imply that I was immediately successful at it. More often than not, during the first years of lupus, I submitted to depression. After all, it was far easier to give in to it than to resist.

During these difficult times I realized I was fighting two wars: one of the body, the other of the mind; yet they were really one and the same—Lupus, the wolf. But increasingly I saw that victory over one, temporary as it might be, could mean easier management of the other. By now I was at least aware of the challenge that lay before me. It was going to be the test of my character. Would I succeed in mustering enough spirit to battle my invisible beast—not just once in a clear-cut, final contest, but repeatedly, for the rest of my life? Or would I allow him also to control my heart and soul, now that he had proclaimed himself master of my body? Would I find ways to cope and survive meaningfully, or would I permit my disease to rule my mind?

Awed by the situation, I did not know how to begin to accept lupus. However, I did know that I could not possibly accomplish the feat by myself. Again the feeling of raw isolation numbed me. The wolf had defined his territory clearly. Restlessly policing his physical boundaries, unsatisfied merely to ravage my body, he now patrolled my mind, working his powers on me. In the end, accepting lupus would also require negotiation with the wolf.

CHAPTER FIVE

The Wolf Rules the Pack

*The hierarchical social organization itself reduces
conflict, since each individual knows his or her own
particular place in relation to the focal leader or
"control" wolf.*
—*Michael W. Fox*

Since the day lupus was diagnosed and became part of our family, Steven had faced his own set of problems. Trying desperately to get a handle on my own symptoms and emotions, I was so preoccupied with myself that it took me several years to realize that my husband was also living through a private hell. His problems were very real and demanded attention: for the sake of his inner peace, my health, and our marriage. Increasingly we both noticed how directly Steven's behavior during flare-ups affected me. When he was able to cope, his understanding and comfort helped me concentrate on improving my condition and attitude. But, when he unleashed his emotions and took them out on me, his adverse reactions made me nervous and anxious. This added to my stress and undoubtedly prolonged the flare-ups. So, for many reasons, it finally became important for me to concentrate on my husband, to understand and deal with his problems for a change, not exclusively my own.

As I mentioned earlier, Steven first learned of lupus when he was on a business trip in Washington, D.C. During a break from a meeting he called me at work only to discover that I had unexpectedly taken the afternoon off. He was disturbed because he knew I was to have seen Dr. Jones that morning. Finally he reached me at my parents' house. I told him I did not want to discuss the consultation on the phone, that I would wait until the next day when he returned. I should have known Steven better. He called again after I got home and forced the news out of me. After muttering some words of consolation, he returned to his business meeting, shaken and distraught. Then after confiding in one of his colleagues, he excused himself and headed for the nearest library.

Steven's first impulse, unlike mine, was to learn about lupus. He read as much information as he could find that day, absorbing every gruesome detail, selectively retaining the most morbid facts. That night at dinner he ordered his first martini, a significant move for a nondrinker. He even indulged in a second but sadly discovered that the sting of gin failed to comfort him. Steven's new knowledge scared him so badly that he slipped into complete denial of it. If he had read that lupus could often be mild, was a controllable, manageable disease for the most part, especially with rest and proper medication, that lupus patients could live a long life, his mind deleted such information. Instead, he opted to dwell on the morbid possibilities: that lupus could kill, or at least attack your brain, kidneys, lungs, heart, any organ, in fact. Lupus was nothing short of THE BIG BAD WOLF.

The first manifestation of Steven's denial was his decision that I must be spared the facts about lupus so I would not become frightened. He did not want me to read what this disease might hold in store for me. He went to great measures to protect me, removing what few medical reference books we had from our house, and quickly hiding any articles he came across in magazines or newspapers. Apparently it never occurred to him that I might go to a library myself, or already had. He also assumed that Dr. Jones shared his feelings and would go to any length to spare me. In that regard he was right.

Steven's other method of denial was to avoid any discussion of lupus. When he could see I was bothered by certain symptoms, he was sympathetic and always wanted me to tell him precisely where I hurt. But, once he knew my hips ached or that I had a sore throat, he did not want to hear any details. He was very uncomfortable and agitated if too much were verbalized. The more I observed this tendency in him, the more it fascinated me. On the one hand, he was capable of being extremely loving and gentle when I was sick; but when I spoke at any length about the symptoms, drugs, or lab tests, he became uneasy and changed the subject. I think he was partly trying to get my mind off my condition and on to something more positive. But he was also attempting to deny the very existence of lupus. If we did not discuss the matter, then it simply did not exist and could pose no threat. It was far easier for him to ignore it than to face it, which did not surprise me. After all, the same had been true for me only one year before.

Not only would Steven not talk about lupus in detail, he also never mentioned it to a single person after his initial expression of concern to his colleague in Washington. When I was having a flare-up, he told people I had a cold or a headache. If people asked me about lupus in Steven's presence, he promptly silenced them. I distinctly remember how angry he was one day when he found that a friend of mine had sent me an article on lupus. He grabbed it away from me, saying it was not written by an expert (which it was), and that it was "none of Bill's damn business." Steven's denial of lupus lasted a long time—well over a year. It might have lasted even longer had he not witnessed my own efforts toward positive thinking.

There was a strange contradiction in Steven's denial, however. Whereas he did not want to dwell on the physical symptoms of the disease, he *was* capable of discussing my dark moods, most of which were a direct result of lupus. His attitude toward them was always, first, to try to draw me out of myself. He teased me, tickled me, urged me to talk and share my thoughts. When I did not react—and sometimes he tried for days—he finally said, "All right. I'm here when you want to talk, whenever you can," and then left me to myself. If I brooded too long, Steven sometimes treated me with complete silence, giving me a dose of my own medicine, so to speak, feeling he had to snap me out of it somehow. And occasionally he roared like a lion about how difficult I was to live with—and he was right. But, more often than not, he tried gentle persuasion and offered understanding. He also proposed active diversions such as movies, theater, and dining out. What I found most impressive about Steven was that he never gave up on me. He was not satisfied until he had managed to lure or jolt me out of my despair.

Another contradiction about Steven's denial was that, despite the fact that he would not allow it in the family environment, he pursued a clandestine research of the disease. The new facts he learned created frightening emotions in him, some very much like mine, which were intensified and exaggerated by his denial of his wife's lupus and his inability to express himself. He was afraid my condition would worsen and perhaps require hospitalization or cause organ damage of some sort. Knowing that lupus could be fatal, though rarely, he thought I might die. At this point we were both in our early thirties and just beginning a life together. The idea of separation through death was one to which Steven had given no thought until now. Primarily, however, he was afraid of the unknown. Not knowing what the future held for me, for us, devastated him. He had always counted on good health and a secure future . Now his young wife might become gravely ill or be taken from him prematurely.

Steven worried that he would not be able to care for me properly should I become very ill. He fretted over every pain I felt. He was also now the only breadwinner and presumably would continue to be for the rest of our lives. Fortunately, we were not in a financial situation where maintaining our home depended on two incomes, but this was still an extra burden for him. And, knowing how anxious I was to work, he was concerned that I be able to find a new, rewarding life for myself at home. Steven worried about my loneliness, with which he could easily empathize. As he sheltered me from his own wearing, threatening fears, always strong for me, he too suffered from a self-imposed loneliness. He had no one with whom he could or would unload and thereby relieve some of his anguish.

Steven was naturally disappointed that I could no longer be his partner in sports, but he was more rational about this consequence of lupus. Sometimes he complained that he wished we could do more things together, but usually he rallied and found people to replace me. Still, he was always conscious of leaving me behind, and he worried about hurting my feelings, though at the time I assumed that he never gave it a second thought.

One thing bothered Steven more than anything else. Neither of us realized it until a few years later, when it came up in a discussion I had with Dr. Melchinger. He had asked me to describe my husband. I emphasized that Steven was a conscientious achiever, very active and successful in his career. Dr. Melchinger looked at me pensively and said, "In other words, *you* are his only failure." The truth of this remark stunned me. I went home and asked Steven what he thought of it. At first he denied the perception. "When someone is ill, you don't consider he has failed and hold it against him. It's chance. Something beyond his control has happened to him." But, when I pushed the matter, Steven could see what Dr. Melchinger meant. In a sense I *was* a failure. I had a disease that brought our marriage and our family manifold problems. Something had gone wrong and it was me. Lupus took Steven by surprise, caught him off guard. He had expected me to "succeed" in life, too, and now I was handicapped. His disappointment in me was real, though he knew I had not deliberately created my limitations. It unnerved him that something in his life had failed and could not be programmed into a success. Only once before had he experienced failure, but then he had been able to reverse it.

When Steven was eighteen he learned the hard way the extent to which a man can shape his future. He entered college far more interested in partying than in books. As a result he quickly flunked out. This completely surprised him, for he had breezed through high school. It also greatly disappointed his hard-working parents, who had tried to bring him up with a respect for learning and achievement. Steven's mother was a saleswoman in her family's clothing store. His father was a civilian electronics engineer with the U.S. Air Force at Lowry outside Denver. On the side his father bought and renovated old houses and apartment buildings, which he then rented. He did most of the work himself during nights and on weekends, intent on providing a good life for his family.

Steven knew full well, by his parents' example, that success and a secure future came through hard work. But he was so scared of his parents' reaction to his flunking out of college that he ran away. He literally hopped on a plane to Los Angeles to visit a friend, without telling his mother and father. They finally tracked him down and persuaded him to return home. His "failure" had been such a shock to the whole family that Steven knew he had to turn it into a success, if for no other reason than to please his parents. First he took summer school courses and managed to get straight A's. Then he reentered college in the autumn and, from that time on, never brought home any grade lower than a B. Finally, he went on to get his master's and Ph.D. degrees on full scholarships. By this time, he was no longer doing it just for his parents. This experience made a lasting impression on Steven and molded him into a high achiever, a man willing to work hard for his rewards.

Because Steven had been able to reverse this particular failure, he assumed he could do so again. Not so with a chronic disease. His parents, like mine, had not prepared him for emotional or physical problems: they had instead emphasized a man's ability to control his life. They had taken good health for granted like the rest of us —until the day that Steven's father, at age fifty-two, was told he had cancer and only a few weeks to live. Unfortunately, he did not live long enough to see his son receive his Ph.D. After the funeral Steven returned to school, immersed himself in his studies, and suppressed any emotions concerning his father's death. In general he avoided discussion of the matter. He tried to believe that it would be the last illness he would have to face for a long time, convinced himself that no similar tragedy would befall him or anyone important to him, and continued his life.

The most destructive emotion that lupus aroused in Steven was anger. He was furious that I had a disease at all and still angrier that it was something he could do nothing about. What completely confounded his rational nature, and therefore triggered his fury, was the way in which lupus behaved, or rather misbehaved. Had lupus conducted itself as logically and predictably as Steven wished, it would have been far easier on us both. But one flare-up after another demonstrated the irrational tendencies of the disease. It was not going to be tamed or banished. Neither Steven nor I could control it, nor could my doctors. Herein lay the greatest problem of all. Steven's usual approach to a problem was that, if something were wrong, you righted it. If something broke, you fixed it. Suddenly here was something he could not regulate. He could not spank it like a naughty child and reduce it to an apology. Never before had he met such an adversary.

Steven's very denial of lupus was rational: if you do not mention it, it does not exist; if you do not let Jo read the facts, she will not be frightened; if you do not discuss her physical ailments, they will not be so severe or last as long; if you jolt her out of her moods, her health will instantly improve.

Life was supposed to be a big kick. What happened? Suddenly Steven was forced to face sickness and pain—unpleasant matters he had otherwise managed to repress . Now not only was his wife ill, but his mother-in-law, with whom he was very close, was dying. In both situations he was powerless. His practical ways of looking at life and treating a problem were not working. Never before had anything so boldly defied explanation and rationale. Nothing could be more infuriating to such a pragmatic man.

One of our friends once said, "Steven is the most rational man I know." The summer when we discussed the possibility of marriage, Steven's first inclination was to line up all the pros and cons. He even wrote them down. The assets were clear to him. But he imagined all sorts of liabilities. Perhaps he would not be able to find a suitable job. Or he might get sick to the point where he could not support his family. Maybe we would not be happy together and resort to nasty fighting, a point to which so many marriages seem to deteriorate. Statistically we had one chance in two of molding a successful marital relationship. I spent most of the summer trying to persuade Steven that life and marriage have no written guarantees. You have to take your chances. You cannot predict the future. It was fine to take money, health, and job into consideration, particularly when there was a child involved, but marriage was also a matter of the heart. Where did love fit in? But Steven viewed love, too, in a very practical way: do not mention it until you are entirely sure of it. As a consequence, he was one of the few men I knew—perhaps the only one—who had reached the age of twenty-eight and had never once told a woman he loved her. Happily, I was the first. Once he said it he meant it, and all his controlled emotions of the heart were released. From that day forward he lavished on me more love and attention than I had ever hoped for.

Steven's denial worked best for him when I was relatively well. When I had only minor lupus complaints, I could manage the household chores, and our life was then fairly normal. During these times, he was able to suppress his anger and fear because there were fewer problems to face. In general he was calm and very patient with my moods. When he did not have to worry about a flare-up and its accompanying problems, he was overly sympathetic and solicitous. If I ached, he massaged me, helped me up the stairs, waited on me, and often asked how I felt. Perhaps by fawning over me he thought he could stave off a pending flare-up. At first I was greatly soothed by Steven's attentions, but after a while his behavior annoyed me. He was like a watchdog, guarding what I ate and did, reminding me what was good for me, and what could hurt me. His favorite phrases were "Don't overexert yourself"; "Don't lift that, it's too heavy"; "Don't eat salt, it's bad for your kidneys."

I began to feel like a china doll, even though I realized that his concern came from love. Suddenly I had become more precious to him than before. It was unlike Steven to be so cloying and protective. He did not understand that he was suffocating me. As a result I began to resist his attentions. I started to hide things from him, saying I felt well when I clearly did not, so that he would stop fussing over me. When he nagged me about where I hurt I was evasive, but he usually managed to pry the information out of me. Steven had an obsession about knowing which part of my body was involved. Perhaps, like me, he could deal more effectively with a concrete fact than with ignorance. Once he knew what area was affected, he was pacified and did not ask about it again.

Steven's extraordinary attentiveness to me and my aches and pains continued as long as they were minor and did not last too long. Once I was full-swing into a lengthy flare-up that sometimes stretched into weeks or months, the situation slowly changed. At first Steven remained calm, patient, and comforting. But after my prolonged rest, reduction of activity, and increased drugs, he expected the flare-up to disappear. When I failed to improve after these measures were taken, his rational nature got the better of him, and he would ask questions that had no answers. Why did I still ache when I was taking so much aspirin? How could I still have a fever when I was on a higher dose of prednisone than before? Why was I so tired when all I did was sleep and lie on the couch?

The more lupus defied reason, the more Steven's anger was provoked. Indeed, his rationality and fury were never more evident than during a flare-up. The two traits were so interwoven that they could not be separated. They fed on each other like parasites, transforming Steven's usually mild, unflappable temperament to a state of nervous tension. He was disturbed by what he could neither understand nor control. And he could no longer practice denial. Things were too real, too obvious, and demanded attention. The emotions he had been able to check now surfaced.

Whenever I was sick for any length of time, Steven's approach to me would change. Because he was not yet articulating his fears and anger, he did not know how to handle them, so he took them out on me. Being the closest person to him, I was the most likely victim of his frustration. Steven grew abrupt and irritable, and was easily provoked. Neglected household tasks annoyed him. He wearied of expending so much energy and attention on me and chores around the house. I sensed his mounting impatience when I asked him to do things for me. He began to needle me about unimportant little matters. His face showed strain and disappointment. I soon realized, too, that his anger was more likely to flame when his work schedule was tight—and he usually had numerous deadlines to meet.

Steven's unhappiness with the entire situation was never more apparent than when he walked through the door at the end of a hard day to find me still lying on the couch, right where he had left me that morning. I could see the muscles in his face tighten as he forced himself to hide his disappointment and smile. It was only natural that, after seeing me prostrate for weeks on end, he was desperately looking for signs of recovery. When he saw none, he tried to muster his last ounce of patience as he probably said to himself, "Oh my God, not another day with her like this. How much longer?" And all the while I thought I was so heroic just to be out of bed, dressed, and downstairs!

Steven's other approach during a flare-up, if it lasted too long, was finally to urge me to get out of the house and socialize or engage in some activity. He had waited patiently for rest and medicine to cure me. When all else failed, he resorted again to his rationality and began to inject me with potent shots of positive thinking: "Maybe if you quit lying there and get involved in something, you'll feel better." "Think how well off you are! You aren't hospitalized. You have all your limbs. You can see and hear. You're in your own home surrounded by an adoring family and you're even able to take care of yourself!" In other words, as I interpreted these messages, "Quit feeling sorry for yourself." I think Steven assumed that, if my problems were strictly physical, the medicine and rest would have helped. When they did not, he suspected I was suffering from depression and self-pity, both of which he thought could be alleviated by getting me up and out and absorbed in something other than myself. What he did not realize yet was that I suffered only partially from mood.

Much of my condition was pure physical weakness, soreness, and exhaustion, which would not disappear if I pushed myself into activity. I might worsen if I did so. Steven did not understand the extent to which my body and mind affected one another. Going to a movie might have improved a bad mood, to be sure, but it would also have deepened my exhaustion. The thought of sitting through a show when I could hardly hold my head up, or when I had a fever of 102 degrees, was overwhelming. Steven rationally said, "All you have to do is sit there!" That was the point. I could not *lie down* in a movie theater! We often went round robin on this until, like a martyr, I went to the movie to quiet him, or found the stamina to insist on staying home.

The result of Steven's needling and prodding me to get out of the house was harmful during a flare-up, though I realized he meant well. The last thing I needed to hear when I was in such a condition, when just getting dinner on the table at night worried me all day, was "Why don't you *do* something?" and "Think about all the other people who are worse off than you!" In the future this logic proved helpful and often shamed me out of a mood. But, when I had not yet come to understand lupus and what was happening to my body, when I had yet to define my feelings toward it, these reminders were premature and only annoyed and hurt me. There was no room for such logic in an enigmatic, bizarre disease like lupus.

The result was that I became agitated and nervous, dreading any sort of involvement with Steven for fear it would lead to conflict. I felt guilty when I had to ask him to do so much around the house and worried that my requests would trigger his impatience and anger. My feelings of inadequacy and dependency were heightened. His complaining and nit-picking made me anxious. I listened to him, tensed, but rarely replied, never more miserable than when I was physically plagued, mentally depressed, and at the same time bearing the brunt of Steven's emotions. There was so much in his attitude and behavior toward me that stung to the quick. Because his feelings were still repressed, I never knew exactly why he had changed toward me, why his usual sweet nature was now so curt and abrasive. I told myself it was probably due to the pressure he was under from the many deadlines he had to meet from his various marketing projects and from teaching a hundred and sixty students. But, deep down, I suspected it was because of the duration and degree of my flare-up. I knew how wearing my disease was on everyone in the family.

Because neither of us understood what we were feeling, we never made much progress during those times. In fact, it is quite possible that the extra strain that Steven's moods put on me, and the friction between us, resulted in prolonging the flare-ups. We waited each one out and, when I finally began to slowly recover, we would gradually return to a more normal lifestyle and a gentler way with each other. In time, when my health permitted us to resume our activities and I was able to take over around the house again, we would ease back into a close relationship. The strain and unhappiness disappeared along with the nervous tension and high-pitched voices. Unhappily, however, during these early years with lupus, the periods between flare-ups were mercilessly short. Each time I improved we knew it would not be for long. The respites were fragile and temporary as we waited for the onslaught of the next crisis, trying in vain to prepare ourselves.

The wolf had made it blatantly clear who ruled our pack— not Steven and his rational ways of thinking and certainly not I, the chronically diseased woman who had never asked to be stalked, tenanted, taken over, and hemmed in by physical and emotional limitations. Now, worst of all, where I had hoped to have some control and influence—working through my illness with my husband—I had somehow unwittingly allowed the wolf to govern. He was the alpha of our little family pack, the designated leader who dictated what we could and could not do, when, where, how. His impact was felt even in our behavior toward one another. I began to despair that I would ever get a grip on him.

CHAPTER SIX

The Wolf Tears Up the Place

*In him the man and the wolf did not go the same
way together, but were in continual and deadly enmity.
One existed simply and solely to harm the other.*
—*Hermann Hesse*

I had been brought up in a home where no one raised a voice, where anger was expressed instead by the cold shoulder or total silence, and where I was taught to be a peacemaker. It made me extremely uncomfortable when Steven and I resorted to yelling at one another. We always went to great lengths to prevent open warfare but, after weeks of a flare-up that had tried our patience and tested our endurance, we were pushed to the limit. Our defenses broke down and we flew off the handle, never fully meaning what we said, but never stopping first to think what the effects would be on one another. These heated arguments got us nowhere and brought only further hurt and misunderstanding. Steven, too, was uneasy during these times, even though his childhood had not been quite so peaceful as mine.

One of the first remarks Steven had made when he met me and observed how I interacted with Lisa and my parents was, "I never knew a family before who lived in such harmony. You never raise your voices at each other! You're so considerate of each other's feelings. There's so much love and caring !" I responded by saying we had our share of problems, just like any other family, but that we usually talked them out instead of engaging in battle. We believed reasoning rather than shrieking was the antidote to misunderstanding. Steven's hope for his own marriage was that it could be one of peaceful, loving companionship, like my parents'. When we were not strained by a lupus flare-up, we achieved this. If we disagreed about something, we addressed the problem quietly and reasonably, often managing to find a compromise that satisfied us both. It was the length and intensity of the flare-ups, our being restricted to the house, closeted with destructive emotions we did not understand, that brought out the worst in us. Ironically, we knew these were the times we needed to be the closest.

The one difference between us was that Steven seemed to be able to forget completely the harsh words we often exchanged. He had not meant what he said in the first place. They were just words he had barked at me under severe stress, and they were simple for him to erase. For me, however, being more fragile emotionally, and highly sensitive, Steven's words had an indelible bite. Their echo haunted me even during our good times. I often wondered how much he had meant sincerely and how much he had said due to the circumstances.

Being a man of purpose, Steven was likely to push me even when I was not in the midst of a flare-up. If lupus symptoms were not visible, and therefore tangible, he assumed I was completely fine and could live a totally normal life. However, even when my strength was at a fairly high level, I still had a certain amount of muscular weakness and soreness that seemed permanent. This muscular symptom became a part of my daily life whether or not I was in a flare-up. It was exacerbated and exaggerated when I was sick but then, unlike fevers, rashes, or lack of energy, it did not disappear when the flare-up subsided, it merely lessened in intensity. If I went out of my way to hide my muscular problems, Steven was able to dismiss them. Unless I groaned as I climbed a staircase, he forgot that my upper thighs flamed at the effort and slowed me down. If I did not play the piano after dinner, as is my custom, he assumed I did not want to. He never thought I was unable to play because of stiff fingers or sore upper arms. What was not blatantly apparent was misinterpreted as normal health. Steven required constant reminding of my invisible limitations when I was "well."

One summer day when we were driving to the beach I said to Steven, "I've been considering auditing a poetry class at Yale. What do you think?"

"Why audit it? That's a waste of time. You once talked about getting your master's degree. So why don't you take the course for credit?"

I was devastated. Again he was pushing me to do something of which I was incapable. "I don't have the strength or the stamina to launch myself on a full-time endeavor, you know that. Starting a master's program is a serious commitment where I'd have to show up for classes, take a lot of exams, compete with young, smart students, and write long papers. I can't do that."

"You could do it if you just took one course at a time."

"Look. I just meant to audit the course for fun. I can learn everything the others are learning without having to go through all the exams and papers. And if I don't show up the professor won't give a damn. He wouldn't even be aware of me."

At this point I was trying to rid my life of commitments. It was all I could do to keep up with my family. If Steven were suggesting, in fact urging, that I undertake a master's program, then he did not yet understand lupus and its devious ways.

Steven continued, "I still think you could handle one course at a time. Why don't you at least try?"

"Steven, I can't believe you're pushing me to do something like that when I can never predict my health! You know what I'm like. If I start something I want to do it right, and now I don't feel that I could even get myself to classes regularly."

"I'm sure if you explained your physical situation to the professors, they'd understand and be lenient during your hard times."

"But I don't want that! I don't want special consideration. If I do it I want to do it just like everyone else! I don't want to undertake projects which I can't manage on my own, or which require me to ask favors along the way."

"That's just your pride talking. No one would hold anything against you if you admitted you had some health problems. God knows you could certainly give them clear proof. But you do what you want. Whatever makes you comfortable. I just thought it might be a good project for you to get involved in."

The conversation was hurtful, because there was nothing I would have loved more than to hold down a job or take a master's. But my health stood in my way. I was having enough trouble as it was accepting my limitations. The last thing I needed was Steven pressuring me to do exactly those things I would have liked to do but had to decline.

Steven also pushed me socially. If we were committed to a dinner party and I began to feel ill during the afternoon, I suggested we call our friends, tell them I was unwell, and cancel. Sometimes I even suggested that Steven go alone. Steven would grow impatient and say, "Absolutely not. You're committed. It's rude to call people at the last minute and cancel. It's one thing if you're laid out with a high fever. But you're just a little tired. If you back out all the time, we'll lose our friends." I felt just the opposite, confident that our friends would understand. However, Steven often compromised, saying that we would leave early if I started to fade. The truth of the matter was that, being a person who could get along fine on six hours of sleep a night, Steven could not comprehend the kind of fatigue I experienced. It was completely beyond him. He usually managed to shame me into going to the party. Most often I folded as the evening wore on, cursed Steven to myself, and we made our excuses. And, of course, the entire time we were there, my exhaustion was so evident that I was not particularly good company anyway. Our friends would have been better off without me.

It did not help Steven's predicament that a great deal of the time when I felt miserable I managed to look healthy. This absolutely stupefied him and was part of the reason why he could so easily forget about lupus altogether. I was fortunate that, by controlled diet, I had kept my slim figure. My hair was full and long, the way he liked it. Often I truly seemed fine. Even my doctor sometimes said, "How are you feeling? You certainly look well!"

whereupon I would produce a "shopping list" of about ten symptoms that were annoying me. So, if I tricked my doctor, certainly
I could fool my husband.

In one way I was relieved and happy I could pull this off.
On the other hand it often misled people. Once, when I was at
a party and had run into a friend I had not seen in twenty years,
she said, when she learned I had lupus, "What? But you look so
lovely!" Then she chuckled a little and said, "Why, you don't look
at all like a wolf!" I was partially amused, mostly hurt by this
remark, even though I knew she said it out of nervousness rather
than cruelty. So, if I deceived everyone around me, most of all
I duped Steven, who sometimes, I think, suspected I was exaggerating my complaints. Both my doctors and Steven learned, in
time, that it was my eyes that gave me away. When I was unwell,
they were not bright and clear as usual. Instead they were often
watery, strained, glazed like a misty fog. My eyelids were puffy,
droopy, hooded, and very hard to hold up.

Just after my diagnosis and before lupus reduced our sports
activities, Steven and I took up sailing. After two summers of inten-
sive lessons we bought a twenty-seven-foot Ericson, which we
moored close by in Branford. During the year between our buy-
ing the boat and actually sailing it on our own, my muscular condition worsened considerably. It never occurred to us, however,
that we would have to eventually eliminate sailing. We discussed
it during the winter and decided we could manage if Steven
handled the sails and lines—the heavy work—and left the naviga-
tion and tiller to me. But we had forgotten the power it takes to
hang on to a tiller in a high wind or a strong current, especially
with a boat of that size. Innocently we began our first season of
sailing alone, with a good attitude and the bright hope that this
would be a sport we could enjoy together. It was not to be.

One mishap after another occurred to us that summer which
had nothing to do with my health. Many sailors regale you with
stories of their problems as beginners. It is common to run
aground, pick up a lobster pot, or run out of gas. We did all three

within the first month. We were nervous sailors, and these incidents heightened our tension and made us more cautious than before. We never went out unless the weather was nearly perfect. We memorized the channel markers with dedication and never raised our sails unless we were practically in the middle of the sound, where we could not possibly collide with another boat.

Sailing back and forth between Guilford and New Haven, we never ventured toward the rocks near shore and particularly avoided the Thimble Islands. Constantly on watch for lobster pots, I shouted frantically every time I spied one. I felt seasick if the waves were more than three feet high. Both of us were tense if the winds were over twenty knots, or if the clouds began to look threatening. At this point we headed back to our slip like little pups with our tails between our legs. If we had a "good" day, which in our vocabulary meant a sunny day with light winds and no clouds, we could enjoy a leisurely sail for a few hours.

Aside from the usual beginners' bad luck, it was my muscular weakness that caused us great anguish, endless arguing, and finally brought the situation to a head. If I woke up feeling tired and weak, my instinct told me that we should not sail that day, for Steven would not be able to rely upon me. But he was like a little kid with a new toy. If I timidly suggested staying home, he was so disappointed that I felt pressured and reluctantly gave in. Then he perked up and said, "We won't go far and we won't stay out very long. You don't have to do anything except manage the tiller. I'll do everything else." How could I say no? Momentarily he had managed to put my worries to rest. Out we went, and every single time we did, we found trouble. Weakness often caused me to lose my balance on deck, which greatly disturbed Steven. He had visions of my flying overboard before we even made it out of the channel.

My first job involved guiding the boat out of the slip as Steven handled the lines, pushed us off from the dock, and then scrambled around deck pulling up the fenders. It took good judgment and accuracy to motor our big boat safely into the channel. I was rarely able to manage it expertly. The winds or currents, or both, often tricked me and spun the boat around just a few feet from the dock. Consequently, we were afraid of colliding with other boats. The traffic, especially on weekends, was heavy. Every boat in the marina was lined up in the channel, waiting to go out to the sound. Once we had motored far out, my job was to hold the bow of the boat into the wind, using the tiller, so that Steven could then raise the sails. More often than not, this was an impossible task for me. It was very difficult even on my strong days, not only because holding onto the tiller was hard, but also because the wind whipping into my eyes dried and burned them and I had trouble seeing. Of course if I let the boat veer out of the wind, Steven could not raise the sails.

At those times Steven yelled at me. The expectation of his impatience made me anxious beforehand. I tried holding the tiller between my thighs and using both hands at the same time. But the strength of my legs combined with that of my arms was rarely sufficient to let me do my job. And if the wind hurt my eyes and I shut them, then naturally I could not be sure I was keeping the bow headed into the wind. So, when it came time to raise the sails, I was already a cowering mess, waiting for Steven's first screech from up on deck. Like Pavlov's dog, I was conditioned to hearing a shout and feeling my stomach turn over as soon as I made a mistake. My usual reaction then was to recoil and grow very quiet. Rarely did I find the courage to retaliate. But then again good sailors would tell you that the crew is absolutely never to raise objection to orders from the captain of the boat.

Not only was I incapable of performing my duties as crew, but I also worried about exposing myself to so much potent sun, despite the fact that I wore a hat, light, gauzy outfits, and sun block. I had to use artificial tears constantly because the wind dried my eyes so much. Because I tired easily—from the physical work as well as the heat and sea air—I often had to lie down below deck, hardly an ideal place to revive. If I were already weak, my eyelids drooped and my head throbbed.

I always looked upon our boat as Steven's new toy but also as a symbol for him. Representing masculinity, daring, and courage, it provided him the opportunity to face the elements, let them play with him, but still prove he could remain in control. Although Steven was just as much a beginner as I, and though some of our mistakes were a result of *his* misjudgment, he had the intelligence, stamina, and brute strength to become an excellent sailor. Given the right mate at sea, he might have achieved this. With me, however, we were always fouling things up. I interrupted the plan. I could not be counted on. The boat was turning out to be yet another part of Steven's life that he could not program to his satisfaction.

Our major trauma occurred on a "weak" day, when we should not have sailed in the first place. As usual, I was in charge of tillering the boat out of the slip. The weather was mild—no especially strong wind or current. But I was not in good health. As I steered our boat out, I lost control of the tiller and at the same time had difficulty switching the gear from reverse to forward. The result was that we banged into the bow of a neighboring boat. Steven came to my aid and veered us off, so there was no real damage. But he screamed at me as he had never done before. He grabbed the tiller, guided the boat down the channel, red in the face, seething with anger.

"Goddamn it! What did you do that for? Now just look what you've done! Jesus, you're lucky you didn't hit him harder or we'd be in one hell of a lawsuit by now. Where was your head? That was just so stupid! Even a kid could do this. I do all the hard parts!"

I dissolved into sobs and could not stop crying for hours. Once Steven had composed himself he felt guilty that he had lost his temper. But the accident highlighted our fragile situation. After I controlled my tears, I explained, "I didn't collide with that boat on purpose. Steven, you *know* I don't have the strength to do this. I just lost the tiller. I don't know how. I just lost it."

Steven replied logically, "But there was no wind!"

I finally mustered the courage to tell Steven I absolutely could not be given so much responsibility, particularly when I was unwell.

He needed to rely on someone strong, and I let him down every time. Consequently, I often put us in a dangerous position. Weather, wind, current, channel, traffic, lobster pots, rocks, none of this had anything to do with our problem. It boiled down to *me* and my muscular weakness. It took many arguments and tears before Steven agreed with me. And here we were supposed to be enjoying ourselves! Fortunately, this incident happened at the end of the season, so we did not sail again that year. In my heart I decided that, no matter how much of a stand I had to take against Steven, despite the fact that my decision would bring him disappointment and sadness, I was never going to sail again. But autumn was approaching and it was easier to let the problem lie low for a while, to shelve it until we both found the stamina to face it and bring it to a resolution. Meanwhile, I was thankful that Lisa, away at camp, did not witness our difficulties. By the time she returned, we were back to normal.

When Steven lost his temper with me on the boat, I believe he was finally venting all his pent-up frustration, anger, and fear about lupus. I do not think he was angry only because I lost the tiller. Never before had he demonstrated such fury. For the first time since I had known him, he frightened me. At last he was letting it all out. We did not realize it then, but his outbursts were edging us closer to an articulation of our feelings about my disease.

Finally the day came when Steven pushed me too far. Toward the end of another long flare-up of exhaustion, leaden, sore muscles, dry, stinging eyes to the point where I could not read, arthritis, lack of appetite, not to mention constant bickering and pressure, Steven came into our bedroom one Sunday morning to see if I was awake yet. As usual he had been up for hours, having just returned from jogging.

He leaned over the bed and kissed me. "Morning. How's my girl? Time to get up and at 'em."

"What time is it?" I asked, sure it had to be three in the morning, judging by the way I felt.

"It's ten o'clock already. Come on, kid. Get up and let's have breakfast."

I rolled over and groaned. "I don't want any. Please just let me sleep some more. I'm exhausted."

"How can you possibly need more sleep? You went to bed at eight last night! Pretty soon you'll be welded to those sheets. Now come on and get up and get dressed. It's a beautiful day."

"I don't care. I can't move. Let me sleep. Did Lisa get breakfast?"

"I gave her some cereal and juice a long time ago. She's downstairs watching cartoons. Well, so no breakfast again today?"

"Steven, I'm too weak." All I wanted was to be left alone.

"Well, then, I'll take you out for breakfast."

"Oh, God, that would be worse. Thanks anyway. Can't you just get yourself something and let me sleep?"

Steven had had all he could take of my flare-up and wanted instant improvement. He also wanted my company and his breakfast. "OK. I can manage. But I'll tell you something, Jo. I've just about had enough of this lying around. You could get up if you really wanted to."

This remark irked me. I was not lying around for the hell of it. I felt Steven pushing me again, failing to understand my situation, being selfish. Amazing the kind of strength you can suddenly muster once your adrenalin starts pumping. Furious, my anger overpowering my weakness, I tore out of bed and started for the bathroom.

Steven asked, "Now what are you doing? You're always going from one extreme to another. First you say you can't move out of bed and now you're storming around here like a Nazi trooper!"

"You want your breakfast enough to drag me out of bed? OK. You're going to get it, Buster. *I've* had it too. How come you knew how to cook before we were married and now you can't even get your own goddamn breakfast? I'll make your breakfast right now if that will make you happy. Watch me!"

I slammed the bathroom door. Steven yelled out to me, "I'm not talking to you. You're a crazy woman! Go ahead and get back in bed. I don't want breakfast anymore. I won't eat it if you make it!" He left the room and banged the bedroom door behind him.

That made me so angry I took the bathroom door and slammed it four more times; the molding cracked and the door nearly fell off its hinge. My muscles raged in pain. I was astonished at what I could do.

Steven came back, sure that I had broken the door. "You pull that stunt one more time, Lady, just try it. And get back in bed. I told you I don't want anything from you."

From inside the bathroom I screamed, "You'll eat breakfast if I have to ram it down your throat! You got me up so now the little boy will get his own way." All the while I was sweating, panting, yanking my clothes on.

As I tore out of the bathroom fully dressed, I shot a glance at Steven sitting on the bed, a confused, frustrated look on his face, and my heart beat with a fury I had felt only once before— when my first husband confessed to me his reasons for wanting a divorce. I had managed to throw a full hamper at him. Of course it did not go very far or even hit him since it was so heavy. I accomplished little but looking foolish and scattering clothing all over the floor.

By this time Lisa was shuffling around our bedroom in her robe and slippers. I tried to get a handle on myself so she would not notice how upset I was. I was struck by her attitude. She was clearly amused rather than frightened, finding it funny that Mom had broken the door. Making a few unwelcome remarks like "Mom, take it easy," and "Dad, why don't you lay off?" she retired again to the family room for her Sunday morning cartoons. I thought to myself, "At least *she* seems to have everything under control." Lisa had witnessed some of our fights and obviously had confidence that this one, like so many of the rest, would be short-lived. In her estimation we blew up over nothing—how could breakfast cause such a stir? I was relieved we had not alarmed her.

Ignoring Steven, I stomped downstairs to make his breakfast, all the while slamming every cupboard door as loudly as I could, still breathless, driven by sheer frustration and anger.

Following me, Steven hollered, "I told you I'm not eating a damn thing so quit making such a scene. You've always got to be melodramatic, don't you?"

"Trying to fuel the fires? Just keep it up and I'll throw a little arsenic in here for old time's sake," I barked, as I beat the eggs vigorously, my tongue spitting venom, my mouth agape with flames of fire. I wanted to make Steven feel as guilty as possible so I made all his favorites—scrambled eggs with cheddar cheese and bacon, and hot blueberry muffins. After I made a pot of coffee, I smacked it all down on the kitchen table. Steven was nowhere to be found. I announced that breakfast was ready and he still did not appear. Finally he came in from the family room. He was no longer yelling but he still insisted he was not going to eat.

"Suit yourself. I'm glad you got me up for nothing. I hope you're feeling really good about this." I poured myself a cup of coffee and banged the front door behind me as I retreated to the peace of our woods to sit on a rock, alone, to think and to cry, in total desperation. I was thoroughly exhausted.

This incident was important because it initiated a new line of thinking in me which was terrifying: that maybe I should not try to live within the family circle, that perhaps we would all be better off if I lived alone. Love Steven or not, I should leave him and let him find someone else with whom he could live a total life. But what about Lisa? Where would she thrive best? With a healthy father who was a workaholic and had to travel a lot or with a mother who, though always home, was almost always sick and disabled in one way or another? Leaving a husband was bad enough, leaving a child was an entirely different matter. Could I? Should I?

Steven, meanwhile, knew he was in the doghouse again. When the door shook the whole house, he came outside immediately. I think he was afraid I might walk away and never return. When he approached me, he saw my tears and began to cry himself.

Between sobs, I said, "When is this going to end? I shouldn't be here. You should have a wife who can make your breakfast and keep you company. If I had the money to support myself, I'd go off and live alone somewhere."

As Flannery O'Connor said just before her death, "The wolf, I'm afraid, is inside tearing up the place." *My* wolf was certainly tearing asunder my inner peace as well as my marriage. My comment about living alone deeply affected Steven. I had not said it for shock value: I meant it and he knew it.

"I did it again, didn't I?" he said, tears staining his cheeks. "I pushed you too far, too hard. I don't know what's the matter with me. I just can't stand to see you sick for so long. I want so badly for you to be well. I miss you, Jo." He took me in his arms and we wept on each other's shoulders.

"Please don't ever say that again," he added.

"What?"

"That stuff about going away. Your place is here with Lisa and me. I'm the one who has to change, not you. I don't need anyone but you. You're all I want."

Working myself into a state of agitation, I paced back and forth, not knowing what to do, whom, if anyone, I wanted to talk to, or where I wanted to go. Then I wept uncontrollably again, while Steven held and reassured me.

"Everything will be fine. We just have to work on this together. I have to stop pushing you, I know. I don't know what makes me do it. But you've got to promise me to stop this talk about leaving. That wouldn't solve anything. I need you and I love you and I want you right here with me."

Despite his words of love and comfort, the thought pounded in my head that I had to get away from Steven's constant pushing and relieve him of the burden of a sick wife. This idea persisted. I loved Steven deeply but felt that, by living with him, I was bringing him down. All of our most difficult moments were due to my lupus. I was always ruining his good times and spoiling our joint activities. And how long could I count on Lisa to be amused rather than concerned? I was sure that eventually I would adversely affect her too. Another thought gnawed me: as a caring, devoted mother, I could never leave my child under any circumstance whatsoever.

I saw no end to the repetitive pattern that Steven and I had established over the years. A flare-up arrived, overstayed its welcome, drained me physically, irritated Steven until he pushed and nagged me, I broke down in tears and despair, and he apologized. Would Steven ever realize that I was by nature an achiever and did not need to be shoved into things? Would he ever reach the point where he could leave me alone to determine what my own activities could be? When I was ready and felt well enough, I would automatically self-motivate. He had to learn to accept the sick part of me as well as the well part. During flare-ups he would have to ignore my lack of achievement and see me as a needy patient dependent upon his understanding and support. Outside of flare-ups he would have to learn to switch gears and rely again on my personal powers of motivation and determination. I knew this was not easy. It was almost as if I were a dual personality and he never knew which person he would be dealing with from day to day. How many times would we end up in battles over unimportant issues like social engagements, master's programs, and breakfast? I wanted desperately to restore peace and harmony to our family. More and more I thought the answer might be to take my lupus and run.

But I was suspicious of my wolf. He would follow me wherever I went, in hot pursuit, unable to let go his hold on me. At least if I were alone he could not affect Steven and Lisa. We would live as a pack of only two, and in time I knew he would grow restless again, meddle with my insides, churn up my cells, tamper with my brain. I was willing to do just about anything to spare Steven and Lisa.

CHAPTER SEVEN

The Wolf Moves Over

Around each wolf is an invisible "balloon" such that
every other wolf respects this inner personal space and
will not violate it.
—*Michael W. Fox*

After I had been home for a couple of years, I slowly began to realize that I had made little progress in dealing with my disease. Too much time had passed with too many unhappy days. I still suffered from the same self-pity and fear. My bitterness and anger, particularly toward Steven, remained strong. I felt I had an enormous burden to bear, with far too many problems to cope with all alone. Not only was I attempting to live with destructive emotions, but I was also trying to deal with my various physical symptoms. When these were not problematic, I spent all my energy caring for my parents. There was rarely a respite. I despaired over how long my mother would hang on, for her sake primarily, but for the rest of us as well. The life she was now enduring at her nursing home meant nothing to her. Unfortunately she had just enough mental capacity left to *know* that she was dying, which made it all the harder for her. Being a stoic woman, she said little, just lay there helplessly taking one blow after another with no power to fight back, except her unfailing instinct to be courageous. Anxious and tense much of the time, I knew that, despite my mother's illness, I had to change my lifestyle, make it not only bearable, but fulfilled and worthwhile, for my own sake as well as those around me. For all I knew my mother might live for many more years. I could not stall in one place. I had to move on.

It is hard for me to pinpoint the exact moment when I made my decision to do everything possible to make some necessary improvements in my life in order to live more peaceably with lupus. Ultimately, after wading through the darkness of my disease at great cost to my psyche and the established serenity of my marriage and family, I opted for survival. But I do not believe the instinct to survive meaningfully surfaces without the patient first experiencing the outright terror that disease delivers, without first fully appreciating the panic of waking alone in the middle of the night thinking you are about to die. After you have been there, you begin to question the validity of your life.

Chronic disease demands a creative response if one is to lead a constructive, relatively normal life within the confines of illness. I suppose that at last something that had been lying dormant deep in the cavern of my soul howled through me like a wild beast. In desperation I revolted. I decided I was not going to live this *non-life* any longer. The will, not merely to survive, but to regain a productive life, plus the resilience of the human spirit, finally joined forces within me. After many years of sickness, feeling left out, complaining, I exploded with anger at *myself* for doing nothing appreciable to alter, and thereby improve, my life. For too long I had waited for pills to fix me, doctors to help me, family and friends to sympathize with me, when in truth I knew that no medical miracle was on the horizon. I also knew that no one besides myself could be held responsible for the condition of my life. No doctor, friend, or husband could cure me or repair my life or convince me to accept lupus. It was up to me and me alone. Sick or not I *had* to find a new way to live. It was alien to my nature to give up, to lose control, when I had been so used to managing and shaping my life. I felt very alone, but a challenge lay before me which I finally had to confront. I had to face my wolf and tame him. No longer could I allow him to govern me.

It was natural, I suppose, that my first instinct was to seek therapy. Indeed, it was the only way I could think of to begin to help myself. I knew, through the Lupus Foundation and my doctors, that there were local lupus support groups I could join if I wanted. I had often heard of their value in helping patients through their worst times, because everyone in the group could relate to you, your symptoms, and the problems you faced. But I was reluctant for two reasons. First, I was already frightened of my disease. I thought perhaps that support groups might include lupus patients with far worse cases than mine. Thus, I would become even more scared, coming face to face with people on dialysis or swollen with steroids. Second, conversely, since I was not an extreme case, was not puffed up or red-faced or arthritic to the point of being unable to walk, it occurred to me that some of the members might resent me. Therefore I chose a different kind of support.

I had seen a psychiatrist once before in my life, when I was going through my divorce, and had found the experience powerful and effective. When I told Steven of my decision to see a psychiatrist I could have predicted his response: "A person can handle his own problems if he tries hard enough." He clung to the old dogma that in large measure only people who are deeply emotionally disturbed need psychiatrists. Certainly he did not want to admit that I was emotionally sick. But I told him I could no longer expect my family to bear the brunt of my emotions. I reminded him that I had been trying to cope by myself but that I was getting nowhere; that his patience with me, particularly with my moods, was waning; and that he had even once barked at me to "shape up or ship out." Steven was alarmed and annoyed that I remembered those words because, he said, he had not meant them. Whether he did or not, I took them as a sign of his growing frustration. They were a definite influence on my decision to go to a psychiatrist. Having lost one marriage, I was not about to put my second one on the line, especially since it had such a solid foundation. I pointed out to Steven that he too would benefit from my therapy because, as I improved, perhaps I would be easier to live with.

I began to see a therapist in Guilford that autumn. Steven ultimately approved, but only because he knew I would go anyway, with or without his consent. He remained skeptical but nevertheless respected me for trying to find a new remedy.

As had been true in my past experience with a therapist, the first few sessions were very difficult. To acquaint Dr. Richard Lewis with my background I had to rehash every painful moment. I had to tell him about the diagnosis and progression of lupus and about the toll it was taking on me as well as on my marriage. But, once I had set the stage, we made progress each week. Usually I came away from my meetings with food for thought, feeling highly stimulated and challenged. Often I cried, and sometimes I returned home depressed. In the long run, however, talking over my problems with a professional was enlightening and helpful. It was not easy to reveal myself at first. But once I opened up, my troubles seemed less overwhelming than before. As had been my experience with Dr. Gifford, I began to feel that someone else was in there pitching for me. Dr. Lewis listened and guided me. He often elicited feelings from my innermost soul that I did not even realize I had. My emotions began to unravel and fall into perspective. When I had kept them locked inside me, they had taken on enormous proportion and were therefore far more frightening than they need have been. I grew less lonely and far less fearful. As the months passed, I began to feel better about myself. I saw some hope not only in battling my disease but also, more important, rescuing my faltering marriage.

By far the most critical advantage of my therapy was that it reestablished a line of communication between Steven and me. For the first time in years I wanted desperately to share my feelings with my husband. Through Dr. Lewis I was beginning to recognize the value of open communication again. It was a welcome relief to vent my feelings, rather than holding back to spare everyone around me. Until the appearance of lupus, I had always been a very forthright, honest person. If something bothered me, I was unafraid to voice my opinions. It was unusual for me to hide my feelings: my disease had turned me inward and away from others. I began to realize how much I had missed being close to Steven.

After my sessions with Dr. Lewis, I returned home eager to share everything with Steven. He was not always ready to listen, preferring not to know what had transpired. It was very difficult for him because he remained suspicious about the value of therapy. But I persisted, encouraged by Dr. Lewis as well as my own instinct. Steven had not yet learned to air his feelings, but he did learn at least to listen to me as I exposed mine. Our talks were often painful, but always eventually beneficial. It was hard for Steven to hear out loud the grim facts about lupus, how I felt it was affecting us as a couple, where I thought he was making mistakes in his behavior toward me. He wanted to think our marriage was perfect. I struck nerves many times as I reminded him that we both needed help, and needed to talk candidly to each other most of all. When I asked him if he would see a therapist too, he rebuffed me with a firm, "Are you kidding? I'll get a grip on this by myself."

Over time, however, it became less painful for Steven to listen to what Dr. Lewis and I had discussed. Less painful, I suppose, because it occurred every week, he could not avoid it, and finally it grew more and more familiar. Once he realized that Dr. Lewis and I were not somehow colluding against him, his awareness of my various feelings was heightened. Whether or not he talked to me was unimportant at this stage. He was finally listening and absorbing, a process that aided him in his treatment of me and in his attitude toward lupus. He respected me for reaching out for help and, as time passed, saw the benefits of therapy to us both.

Dr. Lewis performed another function. He, as the objective observer, talked to me about how *Steven* must feel about having a sick wife, what dealing with a strange, nomadic, chronic disease meant for *him*. This was not entirely new to me. I had certainly given Steven's problems great thought before. But Dr. Lewis's reminders concerning Steven's fears and frustrations helped me see my husband in a different light. No longer was he the cool, gathered, rational man, but a man who was vulnerable and terrified in the face of disease, who suddenly lost his calm and control when the wolf sharpened his teeth, a man who was needy and crying out for help just as I was. Of course Steven was trying his hardest to hide such "weaknesses" from me, but Dr. Lewis made me realize they were there, begging to be properly dealt with. Again I was delivered out of my self and laid at the door of someone else's dilemma. As I tried to focus on Steven's problems as well as mine, we began to communicate at last. And, because I was able to unload my burdens on a professional every week, I suffered fewer bad moods and was easier to live with at home. The more I related to Steven, the less I withdrew from him. In the past Steven had often urged me to "get my act together." Now, slowly, I was doing just that. He had not counted on my therapy affecting *his* life, however, and causing him anxiety. Assuming that I would do it individually, apart from him, he never imagined that he too would necessarily become involved, whether he wanted to or not, sharing some of the pain as well as the rewards. He saw in retrospect that expecting me to suddenly improve my mental outlook and the ways in which I coped with lupus, my parents, Lisa, and my marriage, was asking too much. It would take time, and I could not do it alone. I had to lean on Steven. His understanding was essential for my progress.

After all, we were a couple, and my life and his were intimately entwined. We increasingly realized that we had to work together as a team. Not only for the sake of our marriage, but also for our own individual peace of mind, we had to help one another with our respective problems. It was slowly dawning on us that there were *two* of us involved with lupus, individually and as a couple. If we were going to make progress, we had to join forces against this enemy who had so abruptly and rudely entered our lives and strained our relationship. We knew we would not be able to wave a magic wand and make the enemy disappear, but at least we could work together to tame him. Our combined determination and positive attitudes could only help our situation. When we accomplished functioning as a team, the wolf would be outnumbered and become less threatening, or so we hoped.

At the time that I began therapy, poetry reentered my life. Ever since I was a teenager I had loved to write poems and short stories. Whenever I was faced with a problem, I wrote down my feelings. Most of the poems I wrote in college were stream-of-consciousness love poems and not very good. I also wrote some about my sister's death. Then I wrote nothing until my divorce. But the night my first husband moved out, I sat down and scribbled until I was delirious. It was angry verse, but therapeutic at the time. I found I could release all my fury on paper. As my life took shape once more and I remarried, the poetry stopped again. It seemed to emerge mostly when I was depressed or angry.

Now, with the appearance of lupus in my life, I was facing another trauma. Poetry predictably resurfaced and flowed, almost like automatic writing. At first I wrote primarily about my physical symptoms. Phyllis Rose, referring to George Eliot, said, "In her bargain with life, the body's humiliation was the soul's enrichment; one prospered at the other's expense." So it was with me. If the wolf was violating my body, he was also now beginning to enrich my soul. Gradually I also wrote about the emotional problems lupus brought me—the hurt at being left behind, the deep longing to be included, my yearning for Steven, and the sense of loss I felt every time he left on a trip.

As I let myself be known more and more through poetry, Dr. Lewis encouraged me to do something definite with it. I had never let anyone read my poems before, so was very reluctant to share them. But one of my high school English teachers, I discovered, still lived in New Haven. She now helped run a small, second-hand book shop and tutored at Yale. I called her and timidly asked if she would read some of my work, criticize it, and tell me honestly if I had any talent. Begging her not to lie, I promised that I could take a rebuke from her better than from anyone else. Within two days after receiving my poems, Liz Tate telephoned to say she was deeply moved by them. She thought they expressed emotion very well and said that I should definitely do something with them. Liz knew a woman who lived near me who was a published poet and teacher. She had already given her my name. Rebecca Newth called soon after and asked me to join her poetry workshop. I explained that I felt very vulnerable, that I would be terribly frightened to let anyone else read my work. She was gentle and kind, but made me promise to try at least a few sessions, reassuring me that all the rest of the people were beginners like myself.

Buoyed by Liz's enthusiasm, Rebecca's encouragement, as well as support from Steven and Dr. Lewis, I tentatively joined the group. Much to my astonishment, I found that my poems were not half bad and that I wrote nearly as well as the others. I lost five pounds, however, before I attended my first class. On that night I shook and became very breathless when I had to read my poem aloud. Complete silence followed, and I thought I would pass out from apprehension about what everyone would say. Slowly I overcame this kind of reaction, but it took more than a year of reading aloud before I could do it with a steady voice and no sweat on my brow.

Rebecca was extremely tactful in her criticism of us and never embarrassed anyone. She deftly boosted our confidence, while always pointing out where we could improve. I began to flourish under her guidance, writing many poems, often in the middle of the night when I could not sleep. Suspecting that I had stumbled upon my vocation, I knew at least that writing made me happy, and I looked forward to the feedback from the group, especially Rebecca. Not only did I write prolifically, I also began to read again, voraciously. I had studied the great classic poets in college but had never been introduced to contemporary poetry. Rebecca was very helpful in this respect. I was suddenly on fire with my new learning and with my improving writing skills. And it was exciting to discover that I could write on assignment—not only when I was depressed. However, most of my poetry continued to address the personal traumas I had faced—the "four D's," as Steven liked to call them: death, disease, dying, and divorce.

This was the start of my writing world without which, today, I could not carry on. I deeply identified with Maxine Kumin when I read her words, "I came to poetry as a way of saving myself because I was so wretchedly discontented, and I felt so guilty about being discontented. It just wasn't enough to be a housewife and a mother. It didn't gratify great chunks of me. I came to poetry purely for self-gratification."

Poetry, like therapy, led me to communicate my feelings with Steven. He had read very little poetry in his life, and mine was a rude awakening. It was so direct and honest that it often hurt, because what came out on paper were my inmost thoughts. They were written as clearly as if I had labeled them like dresses and hung them on a rack for display. No one, especially Steven, could possibly misunderstand me. I did not follow the advice that Emily Dickinson proposed in one of her most famous poems: "Tell all the Truth but tell it slant/Success in Circuit lies." On the contrary, I shot from the hip and told it straight.

Because most of my poetry at this time addressed lupus and its accompanying problems, Steven and I began to make more contact as I increasingly shared my poems with him. Again, he was a reluctant listener at first. Shocked and uncomfortable with my candor, he often tried to cut me off. As with my therapy, he preferred not knowing. But now it was my turn to push him. If I felt something, I wanted Steven to know and understand it. My poetry proved to be a great blessing in this respect. Emotions I did not even realize I had, surfaced and took form on paper, just as they sometimes unexpectedly spoke themselves in therapy sessions.

My fear, particularly during seizures, was undeniable:

Something will break this year
Perhaps a collectible—
   my favorite vase from San Gimignano
   the German clock we carried over the border

or a feeling—
   your understanding
   my spirit

As I do not know where I am
as right inverts to left
words stumble out
   slur on top of one another
whole sentences mean nothing
my eyes read from the bottom up

something I know will break this year

My awareness that the health that was born with me had
abandoned me, robbed me of normalcy, was unmistakable:

I see the trappings of my wolf—
the faint rash he paints on my nose
the flush of brow
marbled finger tips
a strained glaze across my eyes
I need no mirror to remind me
that deep in his lair lie
cells ravaged in self-attack
brain waves   allegro   adagio
blood stream   speeding   drowsing
to the beat of his howl

I examine his traces
the stigmata so glaring to me
yet easily hidden from you who might think
at first look I am sound
my inner workings
metronomic

With an unquenchable thirst to reveal what I had written during the day, I would corner Steven at night and read my poems aloud to him. He often remarked, "I had no idea you felt that way," or "I didn't realize you were so scared." The sharing process had finally begun: I had pulled my thumb out of the dike. Steven's turn would come later.

Just as it became easier for me to talk to Steven about lupus, the same held true with Lisa. For me the disease had lost its mystery and terror through discussion, writing, and confrontation. Therefore, I was less reluctant to talk about it with my daughter when the occasion arose naturally. I found I could answer her infrequent questions without worrying what the consequences might be to her if she were told too much. As I grew more comfortable and Lisa older and more mature, I was better able to admit to her, when I was clearly unwell, that I was having "one of my lupus days." I did not have to detail every symptom for her because, by now, she understood well what a "lupus day" meant. Still, Lisa was too young and preoccupied to give lupus much serious thought. Later, once she was in college, we had a long talk about it. At that time she told me how lupus and my flare-ups had affected her as a child. She told me she resented the situation, not me—in particular the way the flare-ups removed me from her life. After my divorce from my first husband, when Lisa and I had lived alone together for two years, we established an unusually close mother/daughter relationship. Because we were so close Lisa was accustomed to having me right by her side whenever she was in need. She also expected me to be a "normal" mother and perform my duties. Suddenly at times I was unable to meet her expectations. Then she was disappointed as well as lonely. She missed my participation in her life. She also felt helpless and uncomfortable, not knowing what to say to me, how to behave toward me when I was sick, or how to assist me. Although she hid it well, evidently her frustration was high during my flare-ups. Wanting to help me, cheer me up, and demonstrate her sympathy, she was at a loss as to how to express her feelings. As a result she avoided the whole situation by removing herself from me. I must admit, looking back on it now, I did wonder all those times I lay in bed why Lisa did not come in to my room more often to keep me company or "shoot the breeze" with me. I should have realized that my illness overwhelmed her. She was just such a good actress that I never suspected she suffered from so much anxiety. But, of course, that was her intention—to hide her frustrations so as not to worry me. She succeeded.

Now that Lisa herself looks back to her behavior toward me she feels that she was selfish, the typical adolescent worrying more about when she was going to be blessed with her mother's company again rather than how soon Mom was going to feel better. I would say she reacted very normally. Part of the reason she wanted me around so much was to act as her buffer with Steven, who was more often than I the disciplinarian during Lisa's early adolescence. Sometimes I could overhear their disagreements and they unsettled me. I wanted to get out of bed and get down there and straighten everything out. Of course, that was exactly what Lisa wanted, too. But perhaps it was all a blessing in disguise in that Steven and Lisa eventually worked out their differences in my absence. As a result they came to know one another better. Certainly I never viewed Lisa's behavior as selfish. Rather I thought she was a typical child, preoccupied with her own life, as she should have been. The last thing I wanted her to do was hang around me all the time, neglecting her friends and activities.

Dr. Lewis, besides encouraging me with poetry, persuaded me to find a circle of friends, realizing that I was terribly lonely, aware of how often Steven traveled.

One day he said, "You have a lot of resentment stored up toward your husband. Why?"

"We've already talked about all the reasons. That he's healthy and active and loves his work and does a lot of things without me. Why are you asking me this when you know the answers?"

"Because I think we have to talk about the last issue. You're beginning to accept him as healthy because you have occasional well times too. And you know you're grateful for his work or else you'd have financial worries on top of everything else. No, I think you have to realize that it boils down to your feeling abandoned, that he leaves you too often by yourself to tend your disease, Lisa, keep the home fires burning, so to speak. And, of course, when he's away he's doing things without you, right? That's what you resent, am I right?"

"Well, mostly he's working. But yes, he has his good times too. I guess that's natural."

"But his leaving a lot and also his enjoying himself, doing things without you, bothers you, doesn't it?"

"Well, yes! How would you like it? Every time he leaves I know I'm in for a long, lonely stretch. No adult to talk to at night. No one to take care of me if I get sick, not that Steven's exactly Florence Nightingale. Then when he comes home we go through this grinding readjustment because just as I've gotten used to his being away, just as I've begun to savor my independence, in walks this stranger, this man of the world who expects to come home and find everything status quo. It's OK for *him* to go out and do things but *we're* supposed to stay home and stay the same. Usually everything is different. Sometimes I'm sick again or Lisa has some flu or something. But mostly we have problems with my mood. I feel angry and yes, a little abandoned when he leaves, if I were to be totally honest, and invaded when he returns. So what's the answer?"

Dr. Lewis responded, "Since it's work that takes him away I don't see that there's much that you can do about that. And I know you're supportive of his building his own consulting business. So what both of you have to work on is this issue of how to handle the many partings."

"Yeah, whoever said 'Parting is such sweet sorrow'? It stinks."

"The reason you hate it so much is that you haven't yet developed a life of your own. You're far too dependent on Steven. Despite your illness you have to find your own interests so that when he leaves you don't feel so let down and abandoned."

"I don't exactly feel abandoned, because he calls me several times a day, but those conversations are worthless. He's always in a hurry, dashing from one meeting to another, telling me he's only got five minutes. God, I hate that. I wish he wouldn't call at all unless we can have a really legitimate talk. He's always hustling me. He tells me what *he's* been doing, then he asks me how I am and what I've been doing. I start to answer but after a sentence or two he cuts me off and says he's got to go. He gets his time, I get nothing."

"So he's just calling home really to make sure you're OK, not to hear all the details."

"Exactly. When I hang up I feel empty. It's bad enough that he's away but he can't even find time to talk to me!"

"What about at night when he's finished with meetings and obligations?"

"That's a laugh. They work by day *and* play by night. Those groups get together at night and do all sorts of fun things together."

"Like what?"

"I don't want to talk about it."

"Oh, yes, you do. Come on. What does Steven do that's bugging you so much? I know you and your marriage. We all know the rules you and Steven live by. So what's he doing?"

I was silent for a long time. Then I began to cry. The idea of Steven enjoying himself without me was tearing me to pieces.

"Well," I said, between tears, "they go out to gourmet restaurants. That's often where he'll call me from. There'll be a lot of noise in the background so I'll know he's not locked up in his hotel with room service or something."

"Is that what you'd like him to do?"

"Well, no, I don't mind his going out with the group to have dinner, I guess. It's the other things. Sometimes they go to movies, a Broadway show if they're in New York, and once. . . ."

I couldn't control my crying. Dr. Lewis was tearing my guts up.

"Go on," he said gently.

112

"Once they went dancing. They were all in a group and they'd just had dinner. Someone suggested they hit a night club and dance. Steven told me all about it. He didn't try to hide it. He was actually stunned when I expressed anger and hurt about it. It was totally beyond him. I said something like 'You mean I was back here on the East Coast eating hotdogs and beans with Lisa in front of the boob tube while you were dining at a posh restaurant and then *dancing?* And just who did you dance *with?*' He said, 'I danced with lots of people. Disco stuff. All fast. Nothing cheek to cheek so you don't have to be so worried.' I told him I was amazed he'd told me and he said, 'Well, I tell you everything else, why not this? I haven't done anything wrong.' "

"Not wrong, just a little insensitive. He might have gone dancing and not told you. You wouldn't like that either."

"Steven wouldn't know how to do that. He likes sharing with me, especially when he doesn't think there's some big sin involved. But now every time he leaves I have this vision of him bopping around with some blonde bombshell."

Dr. Lewis laughed. Even I laughed a little.

"I feel really selfish about this whole thing. I mean I know Steven's not sitting on bar stools all day when he's away. He's working hard. So he deserves to have some fun when the work is over, right? Let his hair down a little?"

"Yes, I think he does. But I think he has to make a compromise with you and realize that these kinds of things hurt you. He has to learn *how* and *when* to tell you, how to be a little more sensitive to your feelings. I also don't think you should feel selfish. There is a great contrast between your two lives right now. You *are*, without asking for it, the sick one at home, necessarily left out of half of his life. It's adversely affecting you. Perhaps with more awareness on Steven's part as well as his agreeing to call you at night for a whole half hour, minimum, to have a genuine conversation you'll feel better about it. And that's certainly not too much to ask."

When I left that day, Dr. Lewis asked me how I felt.

"Rotten. Like I've spread my innards on your table for dissection. But I also think it's good I got it out. That stuff about the resentment. I guess we got to the core of it, didn't we?"

"Absolutely. And now that you realize exactly what you resent—not just his leaving but his having fun—you know now the extreme importance of finding your own identity and life again, don't you?"

Dr. Lewis and I had further discussions about this topic in weeks to come. He constantly encouraged me to get out of the house when I felt well and do something with friends. They could listen to me too, he said, and could provide diversion. He urged me to spend less time on my parents' needs and devote more time and effort to my own. It was extremely difficult to begin reaching out to other people. I had been a near recluse for years, seeing only my family. We had done no socializing to speak of because I was uncomfortable around strangers. I had let old friends fall by the wayside, due to my family problems and embarrassment about lupus. But I knew that the good friends were still behind me, waiting for my return. Slowly I began to contact them. Many were far away, but nevertheless offered their support through letters and phone calls. I also began to reach out to friends I had made at Yale, having occasional lunches with them. Finding the company stimulating, I was relieved to come out of hiding.

Joining Rebecca's poetry class was a concrete step toward making new friends. And gradually, through Rebecca, I met other local writers who responded to me and included me in some of their activities. I began to attend poetry readings in New Haven and to have lunches and dinners with writers once in a while. These new friends, though they did not realize it at the time, helped restore my self-confidence, self-respect, and dignity. The more accepted I was, the less inadequate I felt. No longer did I think of myself as a freak.

Gradually, I was becoming a member of the human race again and was thoroughly rewarded for it. I was not as embarrassed about my occasional rashes, arthritis, speech or thought difficulties when

I saw that my friends were not judging me by my exterior. In time I stopped downgrading myself and began to see my own worth. The acceptance of me as a person, and of my poetry as well, was crucial at this time of my life. Now I rarely lost my temper because I was at ease with myself. I stopped pitying myself as I got out of the house more often and engaged in social activities. This process of rediscovering my inner peace, however, took a very long time. I did not accomplish great feats in a matter of months. It was a progression that stretched out over a four-year period, as I took one little step at a time along the way toward a more fulfilled and meaningful way of life. I made my new friends gradually, taking pride in each, fostering and nourishing each with care, and felt pleased when I was sought out. When I grew close enough to someone, I was even able to tell that person about my lupus.

Restoring old friendships and cultivating new ones led me to a greater acceptance of Steven. I was not as resentful and envious of him as I got out into the world and began to have some outright fun for a change, which was precisely what Dr. Lewis had predicted would happen. As my own activities grew in scope and demand, I became less dependent, stifling, and clinging. Again I reminded myself that Steven was entitled to lead a normal life that included work *and* play, with me as well as without me. It was not my role in life to flog him every time he had a good time when he was off on a trip. Perhaps he had been insensitive at times, telling me things when I was sick which he should have realized would hurt me, but if he was thoughtless, I had been self-centered in expecting him to live like a hermit. Just because I was sick and had limitations did not mean that Steven should relinquish *his* activities and behave like a sick person along with me. Misery loves company only up to a point. It turned my stomach to think I had tried to restrict my husband's natural inclination to live life to the hilt. Choking and confining another person always works to your own disadvantage anyway. In time that person will buck and demand to shed his parasites.

With my life falling into place at last, I found I had some interesting things to talk to Steven about at the end of the day. No longer did we focus strictly on my medical predicaments. They were often a part of us, of course, but now I added to that limited repertoire conversation about my new interests. When Steven traveled I was far less lonely and bitter, because I made an even greater effort during his absence to socialize with my own friends. As a result, I was better able to greet him happily upon his return. It goes without saying, however, that whatever socializing I did always depended on the state of my disease.

Before I made the effort to get out on my own, I had barely been able to speak to Steven when he would telephone home from San Francisco or Chicago. And, when he walked into the house after a five-day absence, it would take me days to readjust, to accept him back without resentment. More and more I felt the need to keep up with him. This could never be done on an equal basis, I realized, because I had Lisa and our home to look after when he was gone, and because I was often unwell. But I wanted to kick up my heels a bit, to alleviate the hurt of being left behind. When I did so, my bitterness let up. I got to the point where I actually looked forward to Steven's trips. They gave me a little space, some breathing room, time with my friends, and time alone with Lisa too. If I happened to be sick when Steven was away, and could not go out to a poetry reading or a movie with friends, my resentment toward him returned.

There were other reasons why I needed to get out when Steven was away. I think that, subconsciously, I needed to reassert the fact that I was *alive*. There were so many times when I was sick and missed out on the fun that, once I was well again, I had an irrepressible urge to get back out into the world, to shout and laugh and tell everyone, "Hey! Look at me! I'm OK again! I'm still with you!" I had worried that Steven would grow too comfortable with me as the stay-at-home wife. He never had to wonder where I was or what I was doing. Every time he called, I was there. While he was circulating in the busy world of business I was sitting at home eating TV dinners with Lisa in front of "Batman and Robin."

Steven noticed the change in me when he was in California one week and called home several times only to find the baby-sitter there. Due to the three-hour time difference, we did not talk to each other at all that week. At this point I was overdoing it, trying to be out every night, deliberately avoiding Steven's phone calls so that he would wonder where I was. Wanting to keep him on his toes and also retaliate, I exhausted myself. Upon his return, he questioned me immediately about what I had been doing. He was worried, but also very curious. This amused me. I pointed out that he had been too confident with his image of me as the traditional wife, sitting home all the time waiting for him. From now on, when he traveled, I would be out too. Steven and I always had very definite standards and values in our marriage, so there was no misunderstanding about what either of us would be doing. I did not want to worry him, I merely wanted him to view me differently: as, at least occasionally, vibrant, fun-loving, dynamic, and self-sufficient again, rather than always the dependent, static, boring killjoy.

It was also healthy for Steven to see that I could have fun without him as well as with him, that now I had a circle of friends of my own, and that I had the strength of purpose to find my own diversions when he was gone. The traditional male in him wanted me to stay home and wait for his calls. But the other part of him wanted me to stop clinging to him and redis-cover my independence. Now that I had done so, he had to adjust to my new ways. He watched me gradually restore my peace of mind and find acceptance of myself. The more comfort-able I grew within my new role, the less I was inclined to criticize Steven and the better we got on together. His interest in me was rekindled, his respect renewed. Like it or not, he had to admit that my new friends and activities were making a better person of me. As a result, I was again an interest-ing, stimulating wife.

About a year after joining Rebecca's class, I was asked to become a member of another poetry workshop in Guilford. I enjoyed both classes because they were very different from each other and exposed me to a variety of writers. Then came still another opportunity that captured my interest. A small literary magazine called *Embers*, which had been started in Guilford a few years before, was floundering because a few of its editors were leaving for other pursuits. The magazine would not survive unless new people joined its staff. Some of my poet friends expressed an interest in the cause and asked me to join them. Still looking for more ways to fulfill myself, I was tempted. Writing, workshops, and readings had begun to satisfy my creative needs, but I wanted more, especially something that would use my organizational skills. I learned that what *Embers* needed was someone to manage its staff, financial affairs, distribution, sales, and the like.

At first I was reluctant, still uncertain of my capabilities and always afraid of commitment because of my precarious health. But my friends pressed me. Finally I offered my services and liked my work so much that, in the course of a year, I became managing editor. This new volunteer job appealed to me for several reasons. Like the job I held at Yale, this also required efficiency and method. I enjoyed communicating with the contributors and encouraging beginning writers, as Rebecca had once guided me. Each time we published, we held a reading and invited some of our poets to read their work. This provided me yet another opportunity to meet interesting people in the literary world, and sometimes led to lasting friendships. Any time I could not work on *Embers* due to ill health, I could rest assured that the other staff members would help out. They were my friends and well understood my predicament.

My writing and the magazine proved to be "jobs" I could handle at home, in my own time, with the support and encouragement of friends and family. No one put demands on me but myself. I worked at my own pace. Gradually I converted an extra bedroom to a study, installing new bookshelves, bulletin boards, and poetry broadsheets. When I felt well, I retreated there every morning with a cup of coffee and tried to write for three or four hours. If I were unsuccessful, I would read. Usually reading inspired me to write. Otherwise I worked on the magazine. I began to take real pleasure in this new lifestyle. It did not strain my capability. Writing became an appetite that required daily feeding. Finally I woke up in the morning and really looked forward to something. Now I *wanted* to get out of bed, sick or not, to get to my work as soon as I could. Even when I felt ill I pushed myself to get into my study and at least try to work. Usually, once I put my mind to something constructive and stopped worrying about my ailments, I was able to produce. The rewards of writing removed some of the bite of chronic disease.

With a great deal of help from other people, I had finally begun to adopt a different attitude. No longer was I always dreary, depressed, and negative. Slowly I was turning to a positive attitude toward my self, lupus, and life as well. While no one asserts that positive thinking cures disease, at least a bright attitude softened some of my misery and, I believe, made me a more palatable person to live with. The more optimistically I thought, the more hope I gained. I knew many negatives had entered my life to stay. But I was gradually modifying some of them, if not completely reversing a few others, through careful investigation of my options. I stopped dwelling on all the things I could no longer do and began emphasizing those things that I could do. Slowly the negatives made way for some positives as I adjusted my expectations, amended my lifestyle, indeed as I began to incorporate lupus into my psyche. Once I saw some positive elements resurface in my life I learned the greatest lesson of all—that *disease need not always be a negative*. But perhaps the chronically ill must hit rock bottom before they can surface with fortitude and a hopeful perspective.

It seemed as if my wolf was making some space for me, moving over to allow me to expand my own boundaries just as he often defined his, forcing me to make room for him. He never allowed me to forget about him, artful as he was at making his presence known. But he was now more tolerant of my need to grow and learn and feel good about myself again. As I pushed myself back out into life, my wolf accommodated me.

CHAPTER EIGHT

Discovering Common Ground With the Wolf

When she was close to the wolves, she would learn
what they could teach her: loyalty, endurance,
stoicism, and courage, the traits that made
them symbols of survival.
— *Ann Arensberg*

Although I was beginning to feel that I did not need a paying job and an impressive title in order to be secure, my new interests provided titles nevertheless. I often gratefully resorted to them when I was intimidated. Now I could say that I was both a poet and an editor. And, because I believed so strongly in what I was doing, I had the courage to talk to others about it. Now that I had something to say, I was astonished to find that people often wanted to listen.

Part of the reason I was able to face others again was that I was growing less ashamed of having lupus. I don't know exactly how this came about. To an extent it was time. The initial shock was wearing off. Nevertheless, I was still facing it on a daily basis, either through therapy, poetry, or flare-ups, not to mention numerous doctor visits. I began to be very curious about my enigmatic companion. Now, as never before, I wanted to educate myself about the disease. Through my therapy with Dr. Lewis I was coming to know my self, and part of knowing me required coming to terms with lupus, facing its austere realities, the cold, bare realities of living with chronic disease. Lupus and I were one and the same: I realized that we could not be separated. Whether it was the wild wolf on the attack, or the tame wolf who kept me company like a pet dog, lupus was going to be my lifetime cellmate, my permanent boarder. The sooner I accepted it, the better. As Sally Fitzgerald said of Flannery O'Connor, "Once she had accepted her destiny, she began to embrace it."

To the extent possible, I too had begun to embrace my destiny. Not only was I carving out a meaningful new life for myself, but I also began to read extensively about lupus. I ordered all the articles available from the Lupus Foundation and read several books as well. As I gradually came to understand what was happening inside my body, lupus became tangible, and consequently less frightening. The stranger within me was no longer so strange and threatening because I knew more about him. When he behaved oddly, I could read about my symptoms and be consoled by the fact that they were "normal," and that many other lupus patients suffered from similar problems, though no two cases of lupus are the same. Because of my research, increasingly I found I could talk about it; and the more I could talk, the easier it was to face the outside world, to emerge from my shell. My shyness and self-consciousness slowly disappeared as lupus became a household word for me.

Besides sheer curiosity, another reason that drove me to learn about lupus was that frequently I did not understand what my doctors told me during examinations. Try as they might to speak to me in layman's language, their medical lingo often left me numb. I sometimes returned home from visits with them and looked up words or phrases in medical books, the same books that Steven had once hidden from me. Once I began my education, I found I actually enjoyed reading about lupus. Comprehending my doctors was also immediately gratifying. I even began to read thoroughly about the various drugs I was taking. The *Physicians' Desk Reference* became my Bible. Acquainted with each medicine's diverse benefits and risks, I was prepared for varied side effects. This was helpful, because I was rarely taken by surprise. Naturally, I still checked with my doctor if I had an adverse reaction, but I was seldom frightened for the very reason that I was informed.

Through an understanding of lupus came an acceptance of it. I stopped hating and pitying myself. Eventually I was even better able to say the word lupus—and it was less overpowering every time I said it. Consequently, I also began to have a stronger hope for living a long life. I thought less of dying, more of how to survive purposefully. As Nietzsche said, "That which does not kill me, makes me stronger." Acceptance of lupus and its restrictions came painfully and slowly, over many years. It required a great deal of determination and hard work on my part, not only as a patient but also as a person. I had to draw on tremendous amounts of inner strength and resilience. Fortunately, I had many factors working alongside me. My own will power combined with time, new activities, sharing through therapy and poetry, the support of my family, the hard work of my doctors, and education about my disease, to encourage a better acceptance of my fate.

My mother was a great help to me at this time. When I visited her one day near the end of her life, I spoke to her about my struggle to maintain a positive attitude. She gazed at me and then, in a rare, clear vision and voice, quietly quoted Reinhold Niebuhr perfectly: "Give me the serenity to accept the things I cannot change; the courage to change the things I can; and the wisdom to know the difference." Evidently, she used to repeat this quite often to some of her nurses. I was awed. Here was a gaunt quadraplegic who knew she was dying, a shut-in living the remainder of her days in a nursing home, who still recognized the requirements of acceptance. I will never forget that particular afternoon with my mother. She sparked my determination as no one had done before.

As I rebelled less and accepted more, I no longer regarded lupus as my master. Instead, I took it on as a challenge and fought back, holding contests with myself during flare-ups to see how long I could remain patient and calm. With positive thinking, constantly telling myself that I could and would prevail, I found I was now only infrequently depressed. Taking pride in my new strength, I defied lupus to get the better of me. I learned to take the most powerful weapon I had—my mind—and use it to my advantage. And I made sure that my mind was equipped to fight, fortifying it with knowledge of the enemy, arming it with the purpose to survive, never to succumb.

My general outlook increasingly optimistic, I took a new lease on life. Even my sense of humor returned and I could laugh again, not only at jokes but also at myself. Now I wanted to live. And more important, I wanted to live *with* my family, not apart from it. I suspected that lupus was something we could all learn to deal with gradually, together as a family. No longer did I consider running away. I had a renewed appreciation for every good day in my life. Nothing passed by unnoticed. As a result, people became important to me as never before. Each member of my family, every friend, and every doctor took on a vital role. I delved into each relationship sincerely and tried not to take anyone for granted. Too many loved ones had been abruptly removed from me and, in the back of my mind, I knew I was living my own life precariously. Although I was no longer preoccupied with early death, I knew it was a possibility. I wanted to ensure that I lived every day fully, giving as much as I could to my family and friends. As Cheri Register said in her book *Living with Chronic Illness*, "Taking frequent measure of the quality of your life ought to be an obligatory feature of the adjustment to chronic illness."

Now that I had begun to learn about lupus and was not so frightened, and had found a way to articulate my creativity, I did not dread the role of "housewife." Being a wife and mother took on a much greater significance because this function did not interfere with my vocation. I was extraordinarily gratified once I realized that it was possible to combine my roles. In fact, the tables turned completely. No longer did I envy other women their careers. I looked upon myself as fortunate to be able to stay home and give something worthwhile to my family as well as to myself simultaneously. At last I had come to believe that a woman could contribute in many valuable ways other than financially.

For instance, I concentrated more on Lisa. She seemed to need me increasingly during the turbulent years of early adolescence. Because I was there every day when she returned home from school, we often had long talks about her problems, which to her were very important and sometimes quite overwhelming. We also spent much time reading together. This had always been our major interest in common, along with horses. When Lisa was very young I read aloud to her every day. We talked about books a great deal and she took pride in beginning her own library. As her scope widened, I especially delighted in sharing the classics with her, rereading the ones that had been my favorites. I also helped Lisa with homework when necessary, and we played duets together on the piano and violin. We took walks with the dogs, often went shell collecting at the beach, and enjoyed watching football and tennis on TV together. As Lisa's friends and extra-curricular activities took on a greater significance, she did not have time to spend long hours with me. But we were always close. I was, and believe I still am, these many years later, the first person she turned to when she was upset or in need of advice. More and more I realized the value of a close friendship with my daughter, especially when I look around and see how many mothers and daughters do not even particularly like each other.

I devoted more attention to Steven too, once I had pulled out of myself and saw that he had problems of his own. Trying to understand what he was going through was difficult, however, because he was not yet confiding in me. It was vitally important to me that we concentrate on the pursuits we both loved in which I could still participate. Steven understood my need. We increased our trips to cultural events, drives around New England, and browsing in antique shops. Ever since we had lived in Belgium, traveling had been high on our list of priorities. So gradually, we took more trips together, venturing through New England, Canada, San Francisco, and of course, Antigua.

The most memorable was a leisurely three-week trip to Italy. Steven rose very early in the morning while I was still asleep. He jogged through the Borghese gardens just off the Via Veneto in Rome, Le Cascine along the Arno River in Florence, and beside the canals of Venice. When he returned to our hotel we enjoyed breakfast on the terrace. Because my parents had walked me all over Europe as a teenager, I took great delight in reading about the various historic sites we visited, just as I had done with my mother and father. I labored over the plans for each day and read aloud to Steven about the places we would go. His interest was usually sparked enough to do some further reading on his own. I did not mind his jogging, because he returned to spend the rest of the day with me.

The more I began to share with Steven and Lisa, the less I resented their activities without me. It was never easy to let them go, but I learned to turn to my own interests while they were gone. Even so, I discovered a definite flaw in my character which took several years to overcome. I did not mind Steven jogging or skiing with Lisa, but if he met other interesting people along the way, replacements, so to speak, I was instantly jealous. This tendency lessened as I found friends of my own and developed a greater confidence in myself. Over the years, as I was accepted and respected by my peers, and as Steven turned to me ever more for companionship and advice, I was not as suspicious and intolerant of strangers. Diseased or not, I now felt that I could make positive contributions to Steven's and Lisa's lives, that they needed me and looked to me for guidance, even if they did not always show it.

Involving myself more with my family and taking on new projects lured me out of my self-preoccupation. Giving more to others, I liked myself better. After I had had lupus a while, I found that it brought me a lot of attention. Strangers as well as friends were concerned about my health, doctors and nurses fussed over me, and my family tended to treat me as a fragile being. Before I realized it, I felt special. But I knew I was special to them in large part because I was sick. A great amount of selflessness and consideration of others is required in a family situation. I did not want to upset the balance, receiving extra amounts of attention just because I had a disease. This, I knew, would lead to self-centeredness. Nevertheless, it was an easy trap and I had fallen into it without knowing it.

As I slowly became a part of the world again, even my doctors took on a greater importance. Increasingly, I deeply cared about my relationships with them. I did not want to be just another sick body to them. Because I was beginning to allow myself to be more fully known to those around me, I wanted my doctors to know me too—how I spent my time, what was important to me, what I felt, thought, dreamed, hoped, or feared. I thought it was necessary that they see Joanna the whole person, not just Joanna the sick patient. They already respected me for learning about my disease, for being informed and cooperative. But they did not yet know me as an individual. I decided to spend a few hours with each doctor, acquainting him with my interests. As I described to each one my aspirations to be a writer and my work with *Embers,* he began to view me as more than a wife and mother at home coping with lupus. Our talks helped them become more sensitive to my needs and feelings. All of them encouraged my newfound activities.

Now I looked forward to seeing my doctors, even if I suspected they might have bad news for me. I was able to talk with them on a personal level, if I needed, and I could joke with them or bring them a gift to show my appreciation. They asked about my writing, my travels, Lisa's school. Dr. Gifford always inquired about my marriage, as I had confided Steven's and my troubles to him periodically. I was especially happy when they chose to tell me a little about themselves or their families, because it enabled me to see *them* as individuals and not just doctors. I was greatly indebted to such caring men, quite aside from the medical expertise they offered me. Consequently, I tried hard to be considerate as well as obedient, following my medical instructions to the letter. I had often seen my doctors exasperated over my condition when they could not help me. Dr. Gifford once said to me, "I really care about you. I don't like it when you don't feel well." Aware of their frustration, I tried not to call unless it was absolutely necessary. Often I had physical complaints but did not tell them because I knew there was little they could do. If, over all my years with lupus, I had called them each time I felt an ache or a pain I would have had them on the telephone daily. I also tried to spare them my depression, realizing that, if I called, it would be just one more burden for them, and it was really up to me to resolve it anyway. Just knowing that I *could* turn to any of my doctors, and that they would caringly respond, was reassuring to me and alleviated my sense of aloneness.

Now that I had made some progress in handling lupus, the battle that remained was helping Steven to find his own ways of coping with the disease and with me. We both knew that he had yet to adjust and accept fate as I finally had done. It was going to be a long, difficult endeavor, considering Steven's rationality and resistance to change. But I was not going to give up on him, just as he had never given up on me. I would be there for him offering all the support I could muster.

Whereas I had begun to "embrace" lupus very gradually, Steven was brought to a heady, rude confrontation with the reality of it. He had rather successfully suppressed his feelings about lupus for well over two years, when his various means of denial were at last flushed out into the open and smashed within a matter of one day, by one brief encounter.

Before I had pulled myself together, Steven had continued to push me socially despite the fact that I had mentioned leaving home. He no more thought I would actually pack my bags than he believed the world was flat. As a result, he managed to remain blind to my increasing unhappiness in his approach to me. There was a cumulative effect to his badgering. As if the summer of sailing and its heated arguments had not been enough, the autumn brought one social engagement after another with which I was unable to cope.

One morning after one such party, when Steven had left for work, I found myself pacing my study, rubbing my hands together, crying uncontrollably. I did not have the vaguest idea what I wanted to do. Part of me still considered running away. Yet my deeply rooted instincts told me that that was not the answer— that problems run away with you. Furthermore, I loved my husband very much and wanted nothing more than to work things out. And certainly I did not want to leave Lisa. Mechanically, I picked up the phone and called Dr. Gifford, who just happened to be in his office. Immediately sensing that I was terribly distraught, he encouraged me to tell him my problems. I poured my heart out to him for almost an hour. Dr. Gifford's soothing voice and understanding reaction calmed me. It had been a long time since he had met Steven, during my initial medical consultation, and had talked with him. He concluded that it might be helpful if he spoke with Steven again and tried to explain lupus more carefully to him. I agreed, saying that if he could not get through to Steven, I would have to consider living alone. Dr. Gifford was surprised when I said this, but I told him that Steven's pushing was tearing me apart and that I could no longer handle it.

Dr. Gifford called Steven at his office and asked him to meet him at the hospital at the end of the day. I took the phone off the hook, wanting to avoid confrontation with Steven until Dr. Gifford had had his say. Nervous and anxious all day, I knew that in Steven's mind, telling my doctor that I was thinking of running away would be a betrayal of marital trust. He would be ashamed and embarrassed, but he might also be angry. He would come away either with a better understanding of me, ready to start fresh, or he would barge through the door, hurt and steaming. I had no idea what to expect.

Dr. Gifford and Steven talked for nearly two hours that November afternoon. The doctor reviewed all the facts about lupus—the inner workings of my body and what went wrong with it during flare-ups. At these times, Dr. Gifford said, Steven's behavior toward me was extremely important: it could either help me improve or worsen my condition. He described once again how emotional stress could trigger flare-ups, pointing out that when

I said I could not handle something, I should be believed. I was not a hypochondriac. I was neither faking nor exaggerating nor pitying myself, merely judging what my body was capable of at any given time.

Dr. Gifford emphasized that I was already highly motivated and, if anything, needed Steven to hold me back and make me rest more. The last thing I needed was to be pushed. It only served to frustrate me and heighten my feelings of inadequacy. Even if I looked well, Steven must remember that I might feel terrible, that it was in my nature to try to spare him and hide the truth. Steven must learn to have confidence in my judgment. After all, Dr. Gifford continued, I was trying to put my life back together again. I needed all the help and encouragement from my family that I could get. He also stressed that it took courage for me to say, "I can't do that," when I desperately wanted to please, participate, be involved, and when the last thing I wanted to do was disappoint my family and friends.

The doctor impressed upon Steven the fact that I had a certain amount of muscular soreness and weakness and a lot of fatigue all the time, whether or not I was in a flare-up. These were my major symptoms, and therefore they were the ones Steven needed to come to grips with the most. This meant curtailing his demands of me athletically. Granted, Steven had already made some progress in this area, but there remained the problem of sailing. Dr. Gifford pointed out that if I had voluntarily given up horseback riding, my favorite sport, I must truly have physical limitations. Steven had not ever looked at it that way before. Dr. Gifford stressed that sailing was especially strenuous and exhausting for me, and that I could not be expected to do anything on the boat except go for the ride. This was the grim reality Steven needed to hear from someone other than me.

I do not think Steven learned anything very new about lupus that day, being widely read on the subject. What the discussion accomplished, however, was first, to refresh his memory, and, second, to force to the surface all the facts about the disease which

Steven had, until then, buried. Hearing the cold, hard evidence about my particular case of lupus from a respected professional had a far greater influence on Steven than reading about it or listening to me. But the real shock of the day came when Dr. Gifford told Steven I was so unhappy that I was thinking of moving out so that I would no longer be a burden to my husband. Steven knew instantly that if I had confided this to my doctor I was serious, and that perhaps he had better take a different course of action with me.

Steven returned home that night a changed man. More gentle and loving than usual, apologetic to the point of tears, he was determined to alter his approach and make everything up to me. Once again we ended up in each other's arms, sobbing.

"I thought you'd be angry with me," I cried.

"God, why would I be angry?"

"I thought you'd resent my turning to Dr. Gifford. But Steven, I wasn't getting through to you. I didn't know where else to go. I was so upset this morning I felt as if I'd do something crazy if I didn't get someone to help me."

"You went to the right person. You know I have a lot of respect for Dr. Gifford. He made me see things differently. Mostly he provided insight. We talked about a lot of your symptoms and how I have to help you more. I have to be more patient and calm, but mostly I have to stop pushing you. I have to trust you to decide what you can and cannot do."

"It's true, you know. You've got to let me be my own judge."

"Well, if Dr. Gifford has so much confidence in you and understands your limitations so well, then I of all people should be able to do the same."

"Steven, all along, all through these years, have you suspected that I was putting you on or something? Exaggerating or faking?"

"Not in general because I know you have a legitimate chronic disease that made you stop working, and I see how sick you are in flare-ups. But there have been times when you look well and you don't seem to have any symptoms and yet you'll still say you can't do something. Or you'll be lying down in the morning telling me how weak and tired you are and then I'll find you out in the garden weeding in the afternoon. That's when I get suspicious."

"Do you understand now what happens during those times? I can look well and still feel some symptoms but I don't like to constantly flagellate you with them. It makes me feel like a whiner if I always tell you I feel rotten. I always figure I'll keep it to myself. After all, it must get depressing after a while."

"Yes, Jo, but that's not fair. If you don't tell me, then I assume you're OK and expect more of you than you can handle. You've got to start being more honest with me. Don't worry. I won't consider it complaining, just reporting, OK?"

"It's a deal. But it'll be hard for me because my inclination is to spare you and Lisa. And as for those times when I'm lying down one minute and weeding later on, you know that's because the weakness and fatigue comes and goes. When it goes away, I figure I'd better use my energy while I've got it because so much of the time I don't have it, damn it, and I never know how long it'll last!"

"I know. I'll try to be better about that. I'm actually glad you called Dr. Gifford. He shamed me into a better understanding of your predicament and my treatment of it."

Steven and I had a long talk that night—our first open, frank discussion about lupus. Steven was still uncomfortable, but I was touched to see how hard he was trying. He was not so evasive and fidgety as he had been before. As we aired a lot of our feelings, I realized that, for a change, Steven was initiating at least half the conversation. With each hour we grew closer. Confronting unpleasant subjects had never been Steven's forte, but the more we talked, the more he saw that discussing lupus was not nearly so painful as he had assumed it would be. When he realized that *I* was able to talk about it, he was able to confide.

Once again we were communicating, and not just that night. We continued to talk, as time passed, about a lot of different things. It was mutually beneficial, albeit painful, as we sometimes tackled delicate subjects. But it certainly relieved a lot of our tension, frustration, and fear, drawing us more intimately together as we drew on one another's strength. We spent a good deal of time figuring out which activities we could increase and which had to be omitted. The boat was our sorest point: we knew that sailing had to be either changed or eliminated. Steven suggested selling the boat, but I feared that he would resent me for it in the long run and, come the summer, would really miss it. I proposed keeping it, but taking other people along with us who knew how to sail and could serve as crew. We could still enjoy the sport that way, but the responsibility would be removed from me. I knew that we had lots of friends who would love to sail with us, who either could not afford a boat or who did not want the commitment of owning one. This is ultimately how we handled the problem, and for a while it worked quite well.

Between Dr. Gifford and me, Steven really had little choice but to own up to the facts and face them head-on for the first time. We eliminated both his methods of denial. He could no longer hide anything about lupus from me, because I had already begun my own education; nor could he avoid discussion about it any more, because Dr. Gifford and I were forcing the issue. Steven admitted as we talked that he felt some of his tension letting up. Witnessing me unfold through therapy and poetry, watching me increasingly adjust to my limitations, encouraged Steven and made it easier for him to follow suit.

After his talk with Dr. Gifford, Steven dramatically changed his approach to me during flare-ups, exhibiting patience and understanding, trying not to push me. This was especially hard for him considering his own powerful inner drive to achieve. It was still difficult for Steven to see me stretched out on the couch for weeks on end. But he restrained himself and I consequently felt less anxious. He began to urge me to rest and take care of myself. When the bad times lingered, I waited for Steven's understanding to dissipate, but he surprised me. He trained himself to outlast me, constantly reassuring me, "You'll make it. Keep up your spirits, kid. You know you'll come out of this soon. You always do. Remember, these flare-ups come and go." His words were all I needed to hear! Suddenly Steven was giving me shots of hope, rather than nagging me and causing me anxiety. Too good to be true? Yes, in the long run it was, but for the time being it was a welcome relief.

My respect for Steven increased. He had seemingly learned his lesson well and was diligently abiding by his promise to let me be my own master. More and more I turned to him for reassurance, feeling safer when he was near, relying on his strength, but also wanting to demonstrate to him my own determination and spirit. Before I asked him to do something for me, I at first *tried* to do it by myself. I wanted to be sure to maximize my abilities as well as my independence. If Steven's new demeanor were only a sham, he was an excellent actor, for I was certainly benefiting from his performance.

Dr. Gifford gave our marriage a great boost. Little did he realize it, but his generous gift of time to both of us and his understanding of our respective problems proved invaluable. During his talk with Steven he had not only explained lupus and my feelings, but he had exhibited a wise comprehension of Steven's difficulties in dealing with the disease and the emotions of a sick wife. Steven did not confide much in him, but Dr. Gifford knew a great deal through me, and in his gentle manner let Steven know that he realized he too was having a hard time. As a result, Steven did not feel that my doctor and I were conspiring against him. He was able to view Dr. Gifford as his own friend and advisor too.

Steven had never realized the vital importance of his own role regarding lupus, nor had he considered how much influence he had on my health. Subconsciously, I think, he always viewed it as *my* disease, and therefore *my* problem. Dr. Gifford made it *our* disease and *our* problem. As we continued to talk, time itself was a great healer. As had been true for me, the initial horror of lupus was wearing off Steven. Over the years my case had remained in control, no major organ involvement had surfaced, with the exception of my psychomotor seizures of the brain, which had proved endurable at least, and I had not had to be hospitalized. Furthermore, my symptoms were no longer strange and terrifying, because we were both growing accustomed to them. Lupus was becoming a household word for all of us. Steven, Lisa, and I often talked about it together. Now a full-fledged member of our family, it was accepted into the pack because stark reality had left us no other alternative.

Steven began to believe it would be possible for me to lead a somewhat normal life after all. Gradually his fear diminished. He worried less about me, particularly as he watched me rebuild a satisfying life. As my interests widened and I did not seem to be hurt at being left behind, Steven could more confidently pursue his sports without feeling guilty. By now he knew that I really *wanted* him to do his own thing because I encouraged him to play tennis or jog. And, naturally, as I grew contented and accepting, I was at peace within myself, far less moody and stormy with Steven, or, to use his word, "feisty." We were beginning to have some fun again, consciously involving ourselves in more activities as a couple. Our "bonding program" had begun, and the results were immediately gratifying. We were close again and felt stronger for sharing lupus on common ground.

Without realizing it, Steven altered his view of me. He no longer saw me—if indeed he ever had—as a failure. On the contrary, he was extremely proud of the way I had tackled my problems and thrown myself into a new life. His own interest in me was revitalized as he saw others accept me. No husband was ever more proud than Steven when I published my first poem. He removed it from the magazine and had it framed. Not only that, he sent me a dozen roses. Steven let me know he was behind me all the way. Whenever I doubted my ability as a writer, he encouraged me. When he returned home from work, he would ask me if I had written that day, even if he was not in the mood for me to read my work to him, which was often the case. This was the man who only a year before had complained that I always wrote about depressing subjects, therefore he did not want to hear about it. Finally he came to see that writing was a purging process for me. Once he understood that it was therapeutic as well as vocational, and that it brought me satisfaction and happiness, he accepted it. As a businessman with little formal education in poetry or creative writing, he supported my pursuits from afar. In truth, he really did not want to have to read my poetry. He did, however, demonstrate his involvement by supporting it and asking about it. That was enough for me. Although I would have preferred he involve himself even further by enthusiastically *reading* my poems, I knew I could not work miracles. This was not his forte, his field, or even his pastime. I contented myself with what he offered me, flattered by his devotion, happy when he occasionally did sit still to read something I had written. I had no idea Steven could care so much about how I spent my time. In his eyes I had turned my "failure" into "success." For him there was no greater reason to lavish me with love and attention. I was doing everything I could to help myself, he thought, and so I deserved credit for my perseverance.

To my surprise, Steven also renewed his education about lupus. Now, when he read about it, he was able to pass on information to me, and this helped to reduce some of the awesome fear for us both. He began to take a great interest in Dr. Hardin's research at Yale. Whenever Steven read about a new drug that might be helpful to me, he called Dr. Hardin immediately to get his reaction. We both began to see Dr. Hardin for occasional lunches, to get to know him personally, and also to discuss lupus and his research in the disease. I volunteered to help with his laboratory tests, sometimes going to the hospital to give him some of what I called "my sick blood" for his experiments. Steven and I together were slowly building a good friendship and rapport with two rheumatologists, each of whom helped us immeasurably in his own unique way. They, in combination with Dr. Melchinger, my internist, formed my essential, dependable medical team.

Over the course of the year after Steven had met with Dr. Gifford, he made extraordinary progress, finally reaching a point where he did not try to hide my disease from other people. In fact, he came full circle to talk candidly about it with others, if the subject arose naturally. Granted, he did not dwell on it for long, but at least he did not appear to be either ashamed or embarrassed. Steven and Lisa came to share lupus in their own way, too. If I had had a hard day, Lisa would clue Steven in when he returned from work. I often overheard them say things like "Mom's having a lupus day," or "It's lupus acting up again."

But though time helped Steven to overcome his fears about lupus, time also began slowly to diminish the impact of his conversation with Dr. Gifford. For a good year it had stuck with him, a constant reminder as to how, ideally, he should behave during flare-ups. Gradually, however, the grim facts faded and escaped his grasp. Unconsciously, Steven began to slip backward, though not to the point where he had been before. He still shared his feelings and talked with me, but I noticed increasingly his old tendency of trying to cut the conversation short when the subject of lupus came up. Understandably, lupus had never been his favorite subject, nor mine, but there were times when we were forced to confront it together. Now he again resorted to saying things like, "OK, I've had enough. There's such a thing as beating a dead horse. Can't we talk about something *pleasant* now?" His impatience took me by surprise. I had been basking in his new-found understanding and was taking great pleasure in watching him move closer toward acceptance of our chronic disease.

Steven's mounting intolerance also became apparent again during extended, difficult flare-ups, when he relapsed into his old habit of pushing me. By now, however, I had progressed to a point where I asserted my rights and thought nothing of gently reminding him to let me be the judge of my own condition. This was usually enough to make Steven back off. But his reversion to former attitudes alerted me that he still retained a certain amount of anger about my disease. This was something I had not considered, for I thought that his anger had diminished. Little did either of us realize that he had merely repressed it again. Although no longer denying the exigencies of lupus, Steven was still fighting it. And, as long as he was furious, he would not be able to acknowledge it completely.

I suppose I had instinctively suspected that Steven's new behavior was too good to be believed. His turnabout had been extraordinarily abrupt. I should have realized that no one could possibly change direction so dramatically without experiencing some sort of falling back. Nevertheless, it was because Steven's progress had been so striking, and had lasted for more than a year, that I was disturbed by his change of heart.

Neither of us understood exactly why Steven began to lose his hold on the situation. To give him all due credit, it was certainly not from lack of continuous effort on his part. Possibly it was because sometimes my condition seemed stabilized. There were many times when I did not feel well, but I was not thrown into debilitating flare-ups either. Insidious symptoms continued to plague me, but I could handle them without involving Steven and Lisa. This coincided with Steven's ability to be concerned but calm. Understandably it was easier for him to be patient when my condition did not substantially affect him. But I, after enjoying a respite for a period of time, eventually regressed into a series of long flare-ups. It was then that Steven's frustration reemerged. He was dependable when I was stable and demanded little attention but, when the true test of his new strength arrived, he was not up to it. When the flare-ups necessitated changing plans, canceling events, or removed me from Steven's company for long periods of time, he lost his grasp. After sticking it out for a few weeks, again my illness defied his reason and he had no tangible way to deal with it effectively.

It was, however, one such lengthy flare-up, combined with other circumstances, that brought Steven substantially closer to "embracing" lupus. Another startling experience shocked him back into reality, but this time, seemingly for good. One summer, right after Lisa left for camp, I became very sick with a fever, burning joints and muscles, and such an overwhelming fatigue that I was laid flat for weeks. My least favorite symptom arrived and stayed for more than a month: my eye glands dried up and the lack of moisture caused me extreme pain. It was difficult to keep my eyes open for any longer than a few seconds, even with lots of squinting and artificial tears. This vastly inhibited my reading and writing—not that I had the energy to do either, anyway. Even watching television was a strain. With no way to preoccupy myself other than listening to music, I became irritable and testy. Summer, even though it supplied intense sunlight, which I had to concentrate on dodging, was the season when we most loved to be outdoors doing things together. But, because it was impossible for me to go sailing or even for a walk, Steven relied heavily on our friends for companionship. Although he never had trouble finding willing partners, he never returned home contented. He always missed me and resented being dependent on others.

This flare-up continued until it was time to visit Lisa at camp. When Lisa had first begun to spend her summers in Maine, we discovered a beautiful resort on Lake Sebago. Rustic yet elegant, set inside a cathedral of pine woods, Migis Lodge offered swimming, boating, water-skiing, tennis, and an excellent cuisine. It was only three miles from Lisa's camp, so Steven would jog over to say good morning to her each day, much to her delight. I *hoped* that I would improve once I changed environments and relaxed in a place where no demands were made on me. This was not to be the case. Every symptom persisted. It was all I could do to walk from our cabin to the lodge for meals, and my appetite was minimal. I sat through most meals feeling sick to my stomach. I could not swim a few strokes without losing my breath, and just sitting on the dock watching Steven water-ski was tiring. Consequently, I spent most of our vacation lying down inside the cabin. Steven, for sheer survival and also, I am sure, to work off his frustration, increasingly involved himself in sports. This effectively removed him from me. The entire Maine vacation was ruined, and it would be hard to say which one of us was more disappointed.

By the time we returned home, the flare-up had been going on for well over a month. Steven's patience and mine were both waning fast. At that time we experienced a two-week heat spell with temperatures in the mid-nineties. Because of my fever I was already hot and uncomfortable, so the extreme temperature outside increased my irritability. Steven was already agitated, being adversely affected by high humidity. He tried to immerse himself in his work, developing his marketing courses for the autumn term and busying himself on numerous consulting assignments.

Predictably, Steven's resentment of lupus began to surface again. He returned home one day harassed and completely worn out. From the couch, trying my best to be cheerful, I asked, "Hi! How was your day?"

Steven sank down in the armchair and snapped, "Hectic, no thanks to you."

"What do you mean by that?"

"I had hoped that you could help me with my work this summer. But I see I can't count on you for *anything!*"

My adrenalin rising to the occasion, I retorted, "Don't you think that's an exaggeration? Sick or not, I still manage to do some things around here, or haven't you noticed?"

"All I notice is you lying on that goddamn couch day in and day out. Isn't it about time you got up and *moved?*"

"Moved out?"

"No, not moved out, for Christ's sake. Just move!" By now he was shrieking at me. "I can't stand it anymore! You've been lying there all summer!"

This reproach was all I needed. I got a nauseating déjà vu from the scene a year before when I nearly broke the bathroom door during our fight over breakfast. I dissolved into tears, an act that normally would have brought Steven to his knees. This time, however, he did not comfort me. Instead, he remained rigid in his chair, a man turned to stone. Looking down between his legs at the floor, he was silent for a long time. I braced myself for the onslaught.

Then finally he barked, "I hate you!"

We instantly looked at each other straight in the eye. And immediately Steven amended his statement.

"Sorry. I didn't mean that. You know that. I meant to say I hate your damn lupus."

Customarily I would have cried more and been terribly upset. Instead, I was gathered enough to recognize great progress in Steven's admission, to the point where I stopped crying altogether. He was at last unleashing his anger: he was letting it all out, and I was relieved. Preparing myself for one of our long, insightful conversations, I said, "Well, *now* we're finally getting somewhere," grinning at him through drying tears. "Say it again."

"What?"

"Say it again! Get it out of your system! Come on. It doesn't bother me. Honey, it means *progress,* can't you see that? Say it!"

Slowly, agonizingly, softly, now looking at the floor again, Steven repeated, "I hate lupus."

"That's not what you said the first time. You said, 'I hate *your* lupus'!"

Steven looked up at me and sighed. "OK. OK, for God's sake. I admit it. I do. I hate it. I hate your goddamn lupus!"

"See what's happening now? You've finally admitted you hate my lupus! We've been waiting for this for years. You hate the disease but you also regard it as *mine.* And it's not! It's *ours, our lupus,* Steven!"

Steven had not seen his comment as holding such powerful significance at first, but he gradually understood what I meant.

I said, "Now we can get somewhere. Now that you're letting your anger out, we can deal with it. Before this, when you locked it up inside yourself, we couldn't get at it. Come on. Let's flush it out and get rid of it once and for all."

Steven came and cuddled with me on the couch. "Do you know how very very much I love you?" he whispered in my ear.

"How do you manage to have such patience and understanding when I say such horrible things to you? I don't even mean them."

"Yes, you do. And it's OK. I used to hate lupus too. And you have good reason to hate it. But as long as you do, you're going to hold me back. I'm trying to accept it and get on with my life. I need you to do the same, Steven."

"I've regressed since my talk with Dr. Gifford, haven't I? I got pretty good at it once. Now I don't seem to be able to tolerate it any longer."

"That's because it never goes away! We never get a break. But you've got to do something, for your sake as well as mine, about this trapped anger you're harboring. It's no help to me during flare-ups, you know that, and it sure puts you in a bad mood at precisely the time I need you most to be stable and dependable."

"Well, I'm always here for you, even if I'm mean."

"I know that."

"You're even the one who has to put up with all the physical problems. I don't even have those to worry about. If we're playing a game here, you're certainly way out front."

"How about if we stop competing and get back to our original teamwork? It's *our* lupus, remember?"

We decided it was time for Steven to aim his anger at a different target. Just as when I had taken out my unhappiness on him years before, being sullen and withdrawn, resenting him, now his anger was misguided. It was unfair for him to constantly unload it on me. Yes, I was the one who had the lupus, but he had to face the truth: that he was angry with the disease, not me. He had to find a way to express his wrath without dragging me down with him. He also had to begin to see lupus as ours, not strictly mine. If we were a team, a partnership, then we shared the good and the bad. Now we shared chronic disease and all its ramifications. It belonged to us, the couple, Joanna and Steven.

Throughout our conversation I took pains to give Steven credit for the other ways in which he had progressed. He felt so bad that I did not want him to be discouraged. I thanked him repeatedly for caring so deeply and for trying so hard. It was important that he should know I was there for him too, just as he had been, always was, for me; that I was aware of the difficult problems he faced. I reminded him that his problems were just as important as mine, reassuring him of my love.

Once Steven allowed his anger to flow, he was able to stand back and take an objective look at it. He could see that it was threatening the progress he had been making, and he definitely saw the negative impact it had on me. Steven earnestly seemed to want to get a hold on his anger. Timidly, I asked him if he did not think that now would be a good time for him to see a therapist, reminding him how much my experience with Dr. Lewis had helped me. I expected Steven to testily reject this proposal. Instead, he said, "I think you're right. I have to do something, though I'm not sure a therapist can help me. I still believe in helping myself. But I know that I haven't succeeded very well, and I'm not doing either of us any good with all this rage."

We both realized that we had shifted positions regarding lupus. In the beginning, when it was first diagnosed, Steven was the one who remained calm, even though his smooth veneer was a result of denial and repression. I was the one who fell into a deep depression. But once I had begun to see Dr. Lewis and had taken decisive steps to alter my life, to fill it out in satisfying ways, I started to improve and, in fact, surpassed Steven in acceptance of the disease. Steven got a late start. He made some improvement with his own problems, but only to a point. He stopped far short of me, and still had a long way to go in deflecting his anger. This was what we both came to realize that summer night. Thankfully, Steven was willing to make the necessary moves to right the situation again and progress even further.

Reluctantly he agreed to see a therapist. He knew I had tried my best with lupus. Now it was his turn. I half expected him to back down, but he kept his promise, only insisting that I be the one to "lay the groundwork," as he put it, with Dr. Lewis. Steven did not want to "go in there and take up a lot of time giving him all the background." I had not seen Dr. Lewis at this point in two years. Steven asked me to keep this matter private between us, because he remained pessimistic and still thought there was a stigma attached to those who sought help from professionals, an attitude he no longer holds today.

I saw Dr. Lewis again a few times, updated him, and warned him of Steven's negative view of psychotherapy. I said, "He's all yours now. Be careful with him and don't offer to analyze his dreams, or he'll run as far as he can!" Dr. Lewis was amused and said he would do his best. I felt he thoroughly understood our respective problems and could handle Steven competently. Dr. Lewis's approach was gentle and easygoing. I did not think that Steven would have any trouble opening up to him.

Steven had only five sessions with Dr. Lewis, but they were enough to get him on the right road again. As had been the case when he saw Dr. Gifford, he realized the value of having a professional help him to see things in a new light. And he was amazed at how easily he was able to talk about his anger and frustration with Dr. Lewis. They discussed Steven's individual problems in handling both the disease and a sick wife, as well as our mutual difficulties as a couple. Each session had its own value. Before an appointment Steven was forced to think in depth about lupus, me, and our situation. He had to get everything fresh in his mind so that he would be able to articulate it. Then afterward, he would come home and talk with me, too. The communication between us was heightened yet again.

Most important, we promised that when lupus got us down, as we knew it would do over and over again, we would scream at it, curse it, hang up a board and throw darts at it—anything but take it out on each other. It was clearly a two-way street. If I did not want Steven to be angry with me during flare-ups, I could not in turn be angry with him for occasionally losing control. We both had to be forgiving and comforting.

We had both learned to cope with lupus in our own separate ways. Now we saw what we could accomplish as a couple.

To vent our anger we took to throwing pillows and magazines, splashing water on each other, slipping ice cubes down our backs, chasing each other with spray cans, and lots of other silly things. Sometimes I would sit down at the piano and pound the keys until my fingers throbbed. I was always ashamed of myself when I did this, having a healthy respect for musical instruments. But I comforted myself, rationalizing that at least it was not a Steinway. Steven often jogged his anger off or smashed it around on the tennis court, much to the chagrin of his unsuspecting opponent.

As we became rather successful at outwardly expressing our feelings during hard times, something else was happening simultaneously. Because so many of our new techniques not only aired our fury but were also funny, we watched ourselves slowly adopt a sense of humor about our disease. We began to see the truth in Viktor Frankl's words: "to see things in a humorous light is some kind of trick learned while mastering the art of living." We invented various ways to make ourselves laugh. When my hips ached and it was hard to climb the stairs, Steven stayed a step behind and pushed me, dramatically exaggerating his huffing and puffing until we made it to the top, both of us in hysterics. When I woke up in the morning so stiff that I could hardly get out of bed, Steven affectionately called me his "tin woman" and offered to get me an oil can, saying, "Don't go out in the rain today or you'll rust!"

I no longer snarled if he teased me about my symptoms, but tried to join in the fun. After all, they were a part of me and I might as well fool around with them rather than merely endure them. In turn, Steven learned to laugh at his temper. One time when he had been especially grumpy, he sent me a card in the mail that said: "GROUCH-OF-THE-WEEK-AWARD Awarded To Steven Eli Permut The First For, By And Far, Being THE Grouchiest Person All Week." We sent each other flowers in reverse. That is, I sometimes had flowers delivered to Steven's office when he had been unruly and impatient, not to reward him but to remind him that, as Horace once said, "Anger is a short madness." Often Steven gave me flowers or stuffed animals when I was well rather than sick. He especially loved to send me little gifts when he was away on trips.

Mostly we worked on surprising one another, trying to come up with new and different ways to give unexpected pleasure. As we expressed our anger and discovered a sense of humor, we found ourselves increasingly indulging each other. This helped to enrich our marital bond and re-cement our friendship. Steven began to leave me notes every day—in the kitchen cupboards, on my typewriter, in my lingerie drawer, even on the steering wheel of my car—to tell me I was beautiful or wonderful or how much he loved me. In return, I baked him chocolate chip cookies, stuck a box of "Good and Plenty" licorice in his Dopp kit when he was about to leave on a trip, unexpectedly showed up at his office to take him out to lunch, or wrote him poems. Over time we gathered a formidable collection of audiotapes of Jack Benny, Amos and Andy, George and Gracie Allen; videotapes of The Honeymooners, Carson Classics, and various comedians like Bob Hope; and books like *The New York Times Book of Cartoons*. Although my "laugh library" was primarily used to preoccupy and amuse me during flare-ups, both Steven and I derived great pleasure from it together.

Talking with a therapist about the disease had a definite impact on Steven, and he was determined to continue his progress—but on his own. He let Dr. Lewis see only just so much of his soul, and no more. His sense of privacy always strong, Steven decided that Dr. Lewis had done his job and could now be dismissed. He was going to take over and manage his own case. To this day Steven has mixed feelings about his brief encounter with psychotherapy. He knows that it helped him articulate his feelings, but he gives most of the credit for this to the two of us rather than to his sessions with Dr. Lewis. It made little difference to me. What I cared about most was happening—Steven was back in control of his feelings and was not afraid to share them with me. Once he was finally able to admit that his previously healthy, active wife now had to lead a different kind of life—but still a fairly normal, happy, and fulfilled life, he was more at peace with himself and, consequently, with me.

Steven's most significant, practical move was his decision that sailing was not an appropriate sport for our family. Because we were growing closer, he had no desire to go sailing without me. He said, "I want to do things *with* you, not without you. I want your company, so why should I bother to pursue something that always takes me away from you?" I found this rewarding, even though I felt badly for Steven that he thought he had to give up something so close to his heart because of me. We were finally on the same wavelength. This was what I had been working toward for a long time—developing and nurturing activities we could enjoy together, not separately, emphasizing what I could handle, not bearing grudges about what I could no longer do. We had named our boat *The Partnership*. When we sold it, we vowed to one another that it was the only partnership between us we would ever dissolve.

Just as the wolf lived with me, I lived with Steven. They both had to share me. And just as my wolf and I discovered a way to coexist, Steven and I toughed out our first years of lupus together, searching for methods to tame the wolf, keep him calm and quiet so that our own lives could be more bearable. The wolf had made his home in me but he had also made space for me. Now he was moving over for Steven too. The three of us had found our common ground.

CHAPTER NINE

Wolf and Patient Negotiate Peace

. . . and even on very rare occasions, they made peace
and lived for one another in such fashion that not
merely did one keep watch whilst the other slept
but each strengthened and confirmed the other.
— *Hermann Hesse*

I was now at a point in my life where I could concentrate on others, rather than on myself. I had moved from self-absorption, from making lupus an all-consuming career, to more involvement in other people's lives. One of these people was my mother. As her condition worsened, it became less important to visit her often. She did not really know the difference, toward the end, between seeing or not seeing us. I tried to conserve my energy, seeing her a few times a week rather than daily, and to make my visits as worthwhile to her as possible. At one time my mother enjoyed my reading aloud to her. But, when she lapsed into a state of semi-awareness, she could not hold a train of thought and found the spoken words more confusing than soothing. She could only lie still in her bed and gaze at me, saying very little. Sometimes she repeated, "Pretty girl, pretty girl," or, "Let me go, let me go," or, "Take me away, Jo, take me away."

When I would talk to her quietly about rejoining her mother and her first-born child, she relaxed and the worried lines on her forehead disappeared. This was my cue that she was preparing herself to die. I emphasized that reuniting with her loved ones again was something she could dream about and anticipate with happiness. Telling her repeatedly what a wonderful mother she had been to me, I often reminded her of the good times we had as a family, and told how I was trying to bring up Lisa the way she had reared me. This was only true in part, since I was in fact trying to be less strict and more openly communicative with Lisa than my mother had been with me. On the other hand, I was certainly attempting to instill in my daughter the same basic values and principles I had been taught as a child. In short, I told my mother what I thought she needed to hear, most of which was indeed the truth. She could not respond, but her eyes were thankful and relieved. I would remain close to her, holding her frail hand, until she fell asleep. When I returned home, I always felt gutted, totally frustrated that I could not do more for my mother. I agonized over her slow death, forever questioning why she had to go so early, knowing how much I would still need and want her in my life.

At last, death was a welcome relief—primarily to my mother, but to the rest of her family as well who felt so powerless and helpless in the face of her agony, watching her gradually, painfully waste away. As selfish as it may sound, I felt a great burden was lifted and a large amount of stress was removed from my life. But so was my mother taken from me, an irreparable loss to me as well as to all who knew and loved her. Aside from myself, however, I was thankful that my long-suffering mother no longer had to face the daily boredom, anguish, and futility of her life and that my sad, despairing father was finally released from his own pain. As time progressed, I missed my mother more. And I felt an overwhelming guilt, always imagining that I could and should have done more for her during her last four years.

My mother's death obviously allowed me to concentrate on my own health again. Attending to my needs manifested itself in many interesting ways. With a growing acceptance of lupus, I realized that I liked myself better. And I decided that that self not only required but deserved some serious physical attention to begin with. Feeling I had neglected my appearance for too long, I first changed my hairstyle. I let the hairdresser lop off the long locks Steven adored and replaced them with a fluffy permanent. Occasionally, I treated myself to a facial massage. I worked on my weight and lost another ten pounds and two sizes, getting back down to what I had been in college. It was important to me to be trim because I could not take much exercise. I wanted to be thin, also, because I knew that at any given time I might have to take large doses of steroids, which would swell my body. Being a little underweight beforehand would give me an advantage, and would also take pressure off my fragile back. Moreover, Steven preferred me thin, and that was perhaps my greatest motivation to watch what I ate.

Clothing became important. I wanted to look good now, for myself as well as for Steven. Even make-up became significant. I had slowly developed a minor lupus rash over the bridge of my nose and was very conscious of it. When Steven called me "Rudolph," that was all it took. I covered the rash with a light foundation cream that I matched carefully to my skin tone. Then came a touch of blush to hide my pale cheeks. Eventually, I tried some lipstick to enliven my general look. Steven was shocked at first, used to seeing me without make-up. In general, he scorned "artificial masks." But gradually, he had to admit that a little color enhanced my looks.

Whereas lack of self-image had previously dressed me in drab, colorless clothing, my new self-confidence was brightening my entire appearance. A friend gave me a book called *Color Me Beautiful*. It described how important it was to a person's general look to wear the appropriate colors, taking into consideration hair and eye color and skin tone. I was disdainful of this book at first, thinking that if I read it I would be taking myself too seriously. But before I knew it, I was hooked. Once I started to read, I could not put the book down. Another friend and I decided to take the one-day course given in our area, and we were "analyzed" by a color consultant. I discovered that I had been wearing the "wrong" colors all my life, tending toward autumn shades like brown, gold, and rust, which made me look pale and sallow. The consultant showed me how much more vibrant I looked in clear, icy colors like pure reds, greens, blues, and purples. This course did wonders for my self-image. It did not make me vain, just more conscious of looking my best—for myself, my husband and even for my daughter, who, as she approached her teens, was beginning to be more actively aware of her own appearance as well as others'. She definitely noticed how people dressed, in particular her mother. What I remember best about the day of the color course is the high to which it delivered *me*. It had been years since I had spent any time on me. And it was fun comparing notes with the other women, helping them muster the courage to change their looks too. My friend and I went out for a drink afterward, then back to her apartment to pick up all the clothes that she should no longer wear, then to my house to sort out the ones I needed to discard. It was thrilling exchanging those clothes, giggling and fussing and rearranging, spending one whole, unspoiled day on myself.

I was interested not only in how I looked. The inner workings and welfare of my body also fascinated me. I began to read articles and books on nutrition, vitamins, and diet. Because I was weight-conscious and usually had little if any appetite, I had developed poor eating habits over the years. For instance, I usually skipped breakfast and instead drank three mugs of coffee, supplemented with aspirin, prednisone, and Plaquenil. I rarely ate lunch unless I went out with a friend, and even then I just picked at a little baked fish. Then I would treat myself to another two or three mugs of coffee and more aspirin in the afternoon. Only around six o'clock did my appetite appear and, more for my family than myself, I would cook a nutritious meal.

I had known all along that so little nourishment and so much caffeine and pills were not doing my system any good, and were perhaps even harming it. My doctors repeatedly warned me that I was heading for a bleeding ulcer, but still I did not listen, being more preoccupied with weight than health. I did not want to eat, but needed the coffee to give me energy so that I could get through the day. What I did not yet realize was that I could get the same lift from natural foods and vitamin supplements, even water, all of which would be far better for my body and certainly for dealing with lupus.

The threat of a bleeding ulcer had certainly frightened me enough to care about what I fed my system. I knew I had to change my dietary habits. After consulting a nutritionist, I first substituted caffeine-free, herbal teas for coffee. If I felt an occasional yearning for coffee, or if I was just plain exhausted and needed the lift to stay awake, I limited myself to one or two cups a day. I began to take multivitamin/mineral supplements and extra calcium daily. In the morning I prepared a delicious "milkshake" for breakfast: a combination of orange or papaya juice, a diced apple or pear, protein powder, lecithin granules, wheat-germ oil, psyllium husk powder, sunflower seeds, a raw egg, and a dash of nutmeg. When I did not feel like something this rich and heavy, albeit healthy, to start my day, I relied on a ready-made protein shake from my health food store which I mixed with skim milk. For something different I had a bowl of Familia cereal, scrambled eggs, or yogurt, adding raw bran flakes and wheat germ to all. For lunch I had some cottage cheese on rice cakes or a small salad, again adding my supplements, always conscious of ingesting as much fiber, vitamins, and protein as possible.

I cut way back on junk food and snacked instead on fresh fruit and vegetables, rice crackers, and nuts; I had long ago completely eliminated salt and sugar. I drank six glasses of water a day, avoiding saturated fats and oily, fried foods. Decreasing my intake of red meat, I tried to eat more baked or broiled fish and skinless chicken. Whenever possible, I ate vegetables raw to get maximum benefit from their nutritional ingredients; and when I cooked them I would steam them lightly and then drink the leftover juices. Suddenly everything I put in my body mattered to me. I even studied medicines and drugs, trying to take only what lupus truly required. I was going to do everything humanly possible to make my body so healthy and fortified that lupus would no longer feel comfortable living inside it. I was going to shock my wolf, make his environment seem alien, and work so flawlessly that he would ultimately reject me in search of another lair.

To this end I also concentrated more on exercise. Whenever I felt strong enough, I either walked two to four miles or swam twenty minutes a day. Of course it took a long time for me to work up to this level of exercise, and it was not always possible due to flare-ups or lack of energy. But when I could handle exertion I built it into my day, also doing sit-ups, leg-lifts, and stationary bicycling at home. A physical therapist helped me design a set of elaborate arm and shoulder exercises to tone and strengthen my upper torso. Again, I was going to make my body so firm and strong that, despite the disease that feasted on my cells, my wolf would feel constricted. Then eventually he would abandon me with his tail between his legs.

I also began massage therapy for many reasons. Primarily my aching muscles and joints profited from weekly massaging. In particular acupressure brought them the most relief, especially in my ever-problematic upper torso area—the triangle ranging from my upper arms, to the shoulders, down to the shoulder blades. Soon my body demanded massage treatment. When for some reason I was unable to keep an appointment, I actually felt stiffer and tenser. I had often heard of the widespread benefits of massage—increasing circulation and flexibility of the muscles, cleansing body tissues, reducing stress, aiding digestion, in short, healing and purging most systems of the body. Before I realized it, I was a convert and a believer. Massage became of vital importance to my well-being.

I discovered meditation in my search for ways to alleviate stress and to remain calm. Not knowing much about yoga or other particular meditational techniques, I turned to the one therapy that had always worked best for me: music. My way of meditating soon consisted of lying down on my bed every morning and every afternoon for twenty minutes each, listening to quiet, soothing, "New Age" music such as Kitaro, Georgia Kelly, and Steve

Halpern. Native American flute music also worked well for me. Eyes closed, phones off the hook, I concentrated on relaxing all the muscles in my body while breathing slowly and evenly. I was able to elicit the effect I wanted and emerged from my sessions feeling at peace inside.

Mental imagery, the conduit between the body and the soul, naturally evolved from my meditation. This entailed imagining a peaceful environment while meditating—in my case it happened to be a meadow laced with red poppies, blue bachelor buttons, yellow black-eyed Susans, with a snow-covered mountain range in the background, a shallow, running brook at its base replete with moss-covered rocks. I would lie in the meadow, my face warmed by the sun, removed from the troubles of the world, at one with nature.

In time I read about visualization, having heard of its benefits to people with a variety of diseases. Patients are encouraged to envision their healthy cells warring against their sick ones. Some, for instance, see vicious, snarling dogs attacking red meat, deriving pleasure from "seeing" their sick cells so madly devoured, believing they will one day recover. One can employ any image as long as it works. What I realized was that in my own form of meditation I encompassed more than just visualization. Not only could I *see* the comforting environment with all its colors that I had created in my imagination, but I could also *smell* the flowers, *feel* the soft grass that I lay on, and *hear* the running water.

****

When I was first told I had lupus, I foresaw only the ruin of my marriage and the destruction of my life. And, quite naturally, when I discovered that *lupus* was the Latin word for wolf, I took an even dimmer and more suspicious view of it. Every image I conjured up about wolves was evil and frightening. Increasingly I associated the disease with the beast. Neither symptomatically,

159

historically, nor mythologically, did I have any reason to look upon lupus or the wolf as anything but terrifying and infamous. And the more he violated my body, the more he provoked my anger and hatred. No one had to remind me that for centuries the wolf has been a symbol for war, lust, deception, greed, savagery, carnage, and witchery. Other animals have been named after the wolf for their predatory ways: wolf wasps, wolf spiders, African wolf snakes, wolf fish, and wolf moths. Killer whales are sometimes called sea wolves.

During the Middle Ages, wolves were hated and hunted. They were considered to be the hounds of the devil, hell-bent on annihilation. Folklore and superstition abounded. It was believed that if a horse stepped in wolf prints, it would become a cripple. Wolves could strike people dumb with their stare, and wolves ate marjoram before hunting to sharpen their teeth. People thought that wolves could be driven off with any kind of music; it was believed that they hated music in general and that is why even today a dissonant note on the violin is referred to as a wolf. Landlords were "wolves," famine was "the wolf," and people who were regarded as werewolves were burned at the stake.

When Christ appeared to Mary Magdalene after the Resurrection, he said, "Do not touch me," or *"Noli me tangere,"* in Latin. These words also mean, in medicine, "any disfiguring skin ulceration, a lupus." Throughout history lupus has been known as "the wolf disease." In the seventeenth century, lumps that might have been what we call breast cancer today were called "wolves," as were sores on people's legs. In the nineteenth century, the lesions of *lupus vulgaris* were said to resemble wolf bites, and the hands and nails of the victims of *lupus erythematosus unquium mutilans* were so disfigured that they were compared to wolf paws.

In World War II, the Allies referred to German "wolfpacks" patrolling the North Atlantic. They called Hitler's retreat in Prussia "The Wolf Lair." Even Hitler's name, Adolf, means "noble wolf."

Today we are "wolfing" down our food if we shovel it in our mouths too fast. If we are in trouble, they say the wolf is at our door. And if we try to trick others for some deceptive reason we are said to be a wolf in sheep's clothing.

The sexual imagery of the rapacious wolf on the prowl has always been pervasive. Most fairy tales tell of the wolf cleverly stalking his prey, be it man or animal. The most chilling story of all is, of course, "Little Red Riding Hood." In the original version, the young girl is followed into the woods by the lusting wolf, who then tricks her into crawling into bed with him just before he devours her. In medieval days, prostitutes were called wolves, the Latin word *lupa* meaning female wolf, as well as whore. And the French have an old expression: *"Elle a vu le loup,"* meaning both "She's seen the wolf" and "She's lost her virginity." Men who want to get a woman's attention often use the wolf whistle, and those who force themselves on women are called wolves.

In astronomy, Lupus, a constellation of 159 stars south of Scorpio and Libra, has long been associated with a beast. Europeans called it the wild animal, and the ancient Assyrians the beast of death. Some thought it should be included in the constellation the Centaur, and considered it a sacrifice, therefore calling it the Victim.

The wolf has been known since classical times to roam at dawn, disappear during the day, reappear at dusk, and howl, unseen, mysteriously, striking terror in the hearts of men during the night. Thus his habits could be likened to lupus, its symptoms coming and going unpredictably, its lingering on the periphery of dawn and dusk, keeping far from the intense sun, and most comfortable stalking the night.

Traditionally a creature of darkness, moving in and out of light, a creature, then, *in transit,* so my own wolf began to transform. As I read more about my disease, so I did about wolves, and consequently my image of them began to soften. Thanks to researchers and writers like L. David Mech and Barry Holstun Lopez, I learned that wolves were sometimes benevolent. To the Romans and Egyptians the wolf symbolized valor. And, if wolves were known primarily as the devil's hounds in medieval times, they were also sometimes pictured accompanying saints, guarding and protecting them. Apothecary shops stocked wolf paws to cure swollen throats, wolves' liver for labor pains, and wolf dung to treat colic and cataracts. In hunting societies such as those of the American Indians, the wolf was revered for his prowess, courage, and stamina, but mostly for his hunting skills.

Over time, wolves were discovered to be caring, devoted parents, both male and female feeding the young. They mate for life, remaining monogamous and dedicated to family life. They kill only when they have to feed themselves, and even then kill old or sick caribou or deer, not because they decide ahead of time which animals to attack, but because, obviously, the old and the sick are easier to catch. Still, preying upon the infirm serves not only to feed the wolf pack but also to allow the fittest animals to survive.

In part due to my reading, and also because I began to recognize that every flare-up had its reward and time of peace, I began to view the wolf differently. No longer was he strictly diabolical. Eventually, the wolf became the metaphor for my disease. After living with him for many years and realizing that at times he was content to lie quiet in the hidden crevices of my body, while at other times he wreaked havoc with my insides, I knew he was there to stay in one way or another. As I accepted lupus, I accepted the wolf. I began to see lupus more as a companion, the enemy wolf changed into a tame pet. He became my life-long tenant, renting body space, and, in an odd sense, he was my ultimate, faithful lover, because he never left me. I could count on him. Even though his symptoms were random and capricious, he was always with me in some way or other, hiding in my blood. Rejection slowly gave way to acceptance.

Predictably, the tame wolf appeared in my meditational imagery. One day, as I listened to the sweet sound of Georgia Kelly's harp and lay relaxed in my meadow, I sensed the wolf lying there beside me, his head leaning on my shoulder, his paw resting on my stomach. Again, not only did I *see* the wolf, I also heard him breathing, felt the flow of his fur when I petted him and the heat of his breath on my neck. Sometimes, when he woke up, he would slowly, gently mouth my limbs.

Now when I meditate, my wolf is always by my side. There are times when he is restless, trying his hardest to be a devil. Then I hear his low growls, and that is when I try to tame him yet again. The wolf image works for me. The metaphor serves the disease, and therefore my self positively. At first I thought perhaps I was weird to spend so much time concentrating on the wolf. But then I read something that Michael W. Fox, a renowned researcher of wolves, wrote: "I often meditate with my wolves and this shared state of being, I believe, involves the collective consciousness of all life and that part of our minds which can connect with others when we cease to think, to intellectualize." The only difference was that Michael Fox meditated with live wolves!

The wolf and I have at last found a way to live side by side without constant combat. I have a collection of wolf memorabilia with which I surround myself: pictures, prints, Zuni fetishes and fetish bowls, Hopi kachinas, sculptures, audiotapes of wolf howls, videocassettes of wolf movies, and lots of books, ranging from myth to fact. In every room of our house there are wolves to remind me of the fragility of my life as well as to serve as my companions.

No matter how kindly I try to view my disease, however, my body remains its battlefield. During flare-ups, lupus and I, intimate though we may be, still war against each other, each trying to gain the upper hand. My wolf is like a twin or soulmate who aches for recognition and competes to get attention when denied or suppressed. But, even when he turns on me and strikes with vengeance, and I feel myself instinctively starting to hate him again, I try to remember that he is also an inner partner, a gift enriching my life in multiple ways. Of course, when I am in a flare-up, it is hard to envision the wolf as my pet. Seeing him rise from his den to attack me, I concentrate on gently talking him out of it, reminding him of how we often get along well together, heeling him to obedience again. It is hard and it does not always

163

work. But once we pull through the flare-up together, I again depend on the wolf to replenish my reserves of courage and perseverance. And, strange as it may sound, I depend on him for his fidelity.

Lupus is sometimes referred to as the great impersonator because its protean, manifold symptoms often imitate other diseases. For me, it proved to be an impersonator in an entirely different way. Unwittingly it acted as an agent of metamorphosis, a catalyst, as it forced me to either drown or surface, edging me from the darkness of disease back into the light of life. I came up with an inner determination and sustenance that I never knew I possessed. An English teacher once wrote to me, after her newborn child had suddenly died of a heart disease, "I have found that nothing is more resilient than the human spirit."

Most important, lupus forced me to come to know and understand who I am inside and out. Then I was better able to accept my self. It led me to richer relationships with family, doctors, and friends, in particular with Steven. Lupus ultimately strengthened and reinforced our marriage. After watching it dip, flounder, sink, and finally resurface over the years since chronic disease stormed into our lives, Steven and I saw that what we ended up with was not what we had begun with. In time lupus brought out our best qualities and delivered us to a level of intimacy we had never known before. Our marriage had grown stronger, closer, nearer to wholeness. Because of living together through years of sadness and stress, not to mention fury and frustration, we had come to know thoroughly every little part of each other. Repeatedly strained and tested, we survived intact with a renewed strength and vitality. Every pain had been worthwhile.

The most important lesson Steven and I learned is that never is only one person assaulted by chronic disease. It smacks the whole family out of its previous life into a new, grim reality—grim until it is understood and accepted. And it shakes up the married couple's bond, throttles it by the neck, threatening to rot its core. Regardless of which partner the disease hits, the other's hell has only just begun. Without continual communication, stamina, and, most important, a positive attitude, the couple will crack into shards of love gone by. The patient stands her best chance against illness when she is reinforced and fortified by her mate. The cold truth is that chronic disease must be a game of double solitaire if it is to be successfully confronted and enfolded into the family.

Ten or eleven years after the diagnosis of lupus I have not only found ways to cope with it, but have come to enjoy my new life. Lupus has worked on my body, but I have learned to combat it with my mind. I am not only surviving, I am happy and fulfilled. No longer do I feel violated by lupus; I am merely inhabited. Strangely enough, I have to admit that lupus has brought many positive things into my life. In addition to a healthier marriage, it encourages my writing, a creativity that would have remained suppressed as long as I worked full-time, an art form that allows me full expression of my feelings and thoughts. I am able to spend more time with the whole family, and I can concentrate some of my creative instincts on our home. And, again, I am involved with other people's lives, which has delivered me from the depths of self-preoccupation. I have now reached a point where I would not trade my new life for my old job at Yale for anything.

Although the battle has not ended, I feel that I am emerging transformed—better equipped to face difficulties in my life, a more secure individual, comfortable and at peace inside. Even when it still terrorizes me, lupus is the greatest journey of my life, a rewarding learning process. It continues to be a broadening experience for both Steven and me as we have learned together that couples can indeed live happily in the face of chronic disease.

I traveled fearfully at first. Then cautiously, respectfully, I moved from a hatred of the disease to an embracing of the wolf.

LUPUS

A disease that can damage any organ of the body can be terrifying to patients, frustrating to physicians, and fascinating to medical scientists. When the cause of such a disorder is completely unknown, and when treatment is not entirely curative, patients are even more frightened. Systemic lupus erythematosus is such a disease.

In lupus patients, some of the body's important defense mechanisms, designed ordinarily to ward off invading micro-organisms, turn against healthy tissues. Antibodies and inflammatory cells mysteriously attack normal organs. Certain parts of the body seem to be more commonly affected than others. It is very rare for any one patient to have all of the problems known to occur, but most patients have three or four different systems involved. Lupus is recognized principally by this pattern of multiple-organ involvement.

For example, the lining of the joints is commonly a site of tissue injury, resulting in arthritis. Lupus is one of many causes of arthritis and joint pains. The skin, including scalp hair, is frequently attacked by the inflammatory process and rashes of all sorts are often found. Hair sometimes falls out in uneven patches. One type of rash is particularly suggestive of lupus and is marked by a distinctive, intense red eruption over the bridge of the nose and cheeks in a "butterfly" pattern. This characteristic facial rash was instrumental in the naming of the disease by an early French physician, who likened it in appearance to the bite of an animal. He called it lupus, the Latin word for wolf.

The disease in some patients may attack normal blood cells and can cause low platelet counts, low white-blood-cell counts, and anemia. In still others, the lungs or the lining around the lungs and heart may become inflamed, causing pleurisy and fever. Fatigue often underlies all of the symptoms and may be the most significant complaint.

When the kidneys are inflamed, the disease can become more

serious and actually lead to kidney failure. Patients are always watched closely for this complication, which may require more aggressive treatment than the milder symptoms of the disease.

Even the brain can become involved. Convulsions or symptoms of profound mental illness can occur. More often, subtle mood changes or depression may be associated with the disease or its therapy. Such symptoms are frequently attributed to other psychiatric conditions, but lupus involvement of the central nervous system may be the cause.

Fortunately, not all patients suffer damage to vital organs. Nevertheless, lupus is capricious in its clinical presentation, and symptoms may come and go without warning. Many seemingly harmless medicines may trigger an attack. Excessive exposure to the ultraviolet rays of the sun can sometimes cause trouble. Pregnancy can intensify symptoms or cause a flare-up after delivery. Unfortunately, lupus is much more common in women than in men and often strikes them during the childbearing years.

Diagnosis of lupus can be difficult and rests with the recognition of some of these typical clinical symptoms, together with the presence of certain abnormal antibodies found in the blood of patients. These antibodies are directed against parts of the nucleus of normal cells. Many types of antinuclear antibodies have been described, but the most serious are those directed against the genetic cellular material known as DNA.

Most patients who have lupus can be managed quite well with current therapies. Many have such a mild form of the disease that they need no therapy at all. Only a small minority have a severe, damaging form. Therapy is designed to reduce inflammation. Full dosages of aspirin remain an important part of such therapy, but occasionally, stronger, cortisone-like drugs are necessary. Rarely, powerful medicines designed to reduce the immune response are employed. Such treatments are nonspecific. A specific cure for lupus must await progress in medical research directed toward improving our understanding of the cause.

— Robert H. Gifford, M.D.

pernicious anemia

Glossary

Anemia — In medical Greek, *anemia* means "no blood." But medical tradition has it mean low numbers of red blood cells, which in turn means low amounts of oxygen carrying hemoglobin, the main chemical of red blood cells. Many illnesses can cause anemia, which then becomes a sign of a disease rather than the disease itself.

Antinuclear-antibody test (ANA) — Some illnesses seem to involve the body's attack on itself. Antibodies against red blood cells are a form of self- or auto-attack that can lead to anemia by reducing red-cell numbers. Similar antibodies helpfully attack infecting bacteria and viruses when the immune system works normally. But when red cells or other normal body cells are subjected to auto-immune attack, we often cannot tell whether the cell became abnormal and somehow like an infecting agent first, or whether the immune system went awry first. Antibodies directed against the nucleus or central part of any cell (antinuclear antibodies) are often a sign of lupus. They may also simply come with aging. There is a simple blood test to determine the level of antinuclear antibodies in the system.

Benadryl — Antihistamines like Benadryl are commonly used to dry nose secretions in early stages of simple colds or allergic reactions to pollens, animal dandruff, feathers, and other irritants. Antihistamines also help control hives, which are swollen, itching red skin lumps caused by some allergic problem.

Central Nervous System Lupus (CNS Lupus) — The brain, in medical parlance, is the "central nervous system." The spinal cord is often included in the CNS, but the peripheral nerves of the arms, legs, and body are not. Lupus can affect the central nervous system or brain at least by inflaming its blood vessels. This may interfere with blood flow to the brain in a very variable way. The brain may then become subtly inflamed itself and thus strangely upset its owner's ideas, perceptions, and movements.

Dilantin — Dilantin is a trade name for phenytoin. This drug is a major chemical tool in controlling psychomotor seizures as well as other types of seizures. There are many potential side

169

effects. The way it works is not at all clear, but, almost by definition, it presumably helps correct the chemical and electrical problems that seem to start seizures in brain cells.

Electroencephalogram (EEG) — An electroencephalogram (EEG) is a graphic recording of the brain's electrical activity. Electrodes are placed on the scalp and are then channeled to an electroencephalograph. This amplifier is attached to a mechanism that converts the brain's electrical impulses to vertical movement of a pen on a piece of paper.

Flare-up — A flare-up is an exacerbation of lupus when all or only some of the patient's symptoms may appear. The duration of a flare-up may range from days to months. It is also common for a lupus patient to experience a flare-up after withdrawal from cortisone treatment or other drugs.

Hypoglycemia — Unfortunately, hypoglycemia, or abnormally low blood sugar, is difficult to diagnose absolutely and is easy to confuse with other causes of fatigue. Ideally, people with hypoglycemia who drink 100 grams of glucose (a kind of sugar) in supervised tests will provoke some symptoms of lip and finger tingling, sweating, fast heart beats, hunger, and confusion as their blood glucose falls dangerously low. These tests last six hours and can be complicated in their interpretation as well as occasionally dangerous. Severe hypoglycemia is rare. Minor cases are difficult to separate from normal.

Lithium — Lithium carbonate still seems a strangely simple treatment for manic-depressive disease. The worst cases are the most dramatic, although the rarest. A severe mania-to-depression swing might find a patient trying to sell the Brooklyn Bridge one week and trying to jump off it the next. These swings are rarely so obvious, but coming and going is their hallmark. Lithium can break the cycles or blunt them wonderfully, if it works.

Lithium toxicity — Lithium toxicity refers to a harmful amount of lithium in the system.

Lupus research — Dr. John A. Hardin, Chief of Rheumatology, Yale University School of Medicine: "Dr. Hardin's research laboratory is devoted to understanding the cause of systemic lupus erythematosus. His approach to this disease begins with the consideration that almost all patients with lupus have in their blood characteristic autoantibodies known as antinuclear antibodies. They are the one common denominator found in this disease, and his research group has reasoned that the process which is responsible for antinuclear antibodies must be closely related to the cause of lupus.

"Normally, the body produces antibodies to protect itself from foreign agents such as viruses and bacteria. However, in the case of lupus, some antibodies are formed that react against the body's own tissues. Such antibodies are referred to as autoantibodies, and when they react against molecules found within the nucleus of cells, they are known as antinuclear antibodies. The strategy in Hardin's laboratory has been to identify the specific molecules of normal tissues that are attacked by antinuclear antibodies from patients with lupus. His group uses the techniques of molecular biology, especially gene-cloning methods, to understand exactly how this attack is carried out. This work has led to the identification of a selected set of molecules which are found in virtually all living cells that have a special propensity to initiate the autoimmune responses of systemic lupus. It appears that these molecules are intimately involved in the early events that lead to systemic lupus. Hardin's laboratory is currently working on understanding exactly how these molecules interact with the immune system in order to learn how to interrupt this process. This information should lead to an understanding of how to stop lupus at the earliest stages of its development."

Mestinon — *Mestinon* is one trade name of pyridostigmine, which increases muscle strength in myasthenia gravis. The drug's action is one of allowing a pile-up of a nerve's chemical signal to its muscle. The excess chemical signal (acetylcholine) activates the otherwise insensitive muscle. However, too much medication makes the chemical messenger pile up dangerously, so an expected toxic effect is too much muscle stimulation.

Mononucleosis — Sometimes popularly called and incorrectly named "the kissing disease" by an Army physician at West Point, mononucleosis is now recognized as a peculiar virus infection often causing marked swelling of all the body's lymph glands. Its reputation for causing fatigue is often overrated.

Myasthenia gravis (MG) — *Myasthenia gravis* (MG) means grave or severe muscle weakness caused by poorly understood defects in muscles' response to chemical messages from their associated nerves. The nerves command, but the muscles hear poorly. MG is a rare but serious condition in which eyelids droop, hips cannot climb stairs, arms cannot comb hair, throats cannot swallow, and diaphragms sometimes cannot breathe. There is therapy, but no cure yet.

Myositis — *Myositis* means muscle inflammation and does not per se suggest the cause. Most chronic myositis has poorly understood causes. Lupus usually causes a myopathy or muscle weakness without inflammation. The same result can also be caused by prednisone.

Neuritis — In medical jargon, the ending "itis" indicates inflammation, a matter of heat, swelling, redness, and pain. Infection need not be the cause. "Neuritis" implies painful swelling in some nerve without indicating the cause.

Plaquenil — *Plaquenil* is a trade name for hydroxychloroquine, used in some parts of the world to prevent or treat malaria. Its chief advantage in lupus control is skin improvement and perhaps joint improvement. Its chief drawback is damage to the retinas, so vision needs regular checking.

Platelets — After white cells and red cells, platelets are the third and smallest particles of blood visible in a microscope. On standard glass laboratory slides, they look like little plates. Platelets are often called thrombocytes to emphasize their role in helping to make clots or thrombi. Their lack can lead to bleeding.

Polymyalgia — Certain overlaps in medical terms are obvious. *Poly* means many, and *myalgia* means muscle aches. This word could mean aching all over and, if you had lupus, could also imply that you had muscle inflammation, or myositis.

Prednisone — Prednisone is one of the common forms of steroids derived from cortisone, the best-known steroid. Cortisone and prednisone reduce inflammation, the normal body's response to any tissue injury. If the inflammatory response is serious and more damaging than helpful, anti-inflammatory drugs like prednisone offer better control than the simpler, safer, and cheaper aspirin. Prednisone, along with other long-term side effects, can cause muscle weakness that affects the shoulders and hips most. Generally, low doses of five milligrams a day do not produce the problem, so lupus itself would be the more likely cause of muscle weakness.

Psychomotor seizures — Psychomotor seizures, now also called mixed motor seizures, are a form of epilepsy, or "fits," where abnormal muscle action is usually mild and periods of confusion are common. Such seizures are also sometimes found in central nervous system lupus.

Raynaud's Phenomenon — Cold skin becomes bloodless. The body thus conserves the blood's heat, but at the risk of skin damage. We know this at its worst as frostbite. Excessive reaction like this in finger tips was described by a French physician, Raynaud, as a sign of some diseases, although it more often occurs as a simple hereditary problem or as a reaction to smoking.

Shingles — *Shingles* is a common household word for what is technically known as herpes zoster, a skin inflammation with blisters and later crusts that give it its name. The cause is activation of chicken pox virus lying latent in nerves after childhood infection. Shingles is usually painful on the chest or the abdomen. It can be devastating in an eye.

Sjogren's Syndrome — Sjogren was the physician who first described the simultaneous lack of tears and saliva in his patients with rheumatoid arthritis. The pattern of poor tear and salivary gland function produces dry eyes and dry mouth. Sjogren's Syndrome now is known to occur in several illnesses or by itself.

Tensilon Test — *Tensilon* is a trade name for edrophonium. It works very much like Mestinon and other medications for MG to amplify nerve signals to muscles. Its brief action makes it good for short tests to see if a patient with muscle weakness gets stronger. If so, the patient *may* have myasthenia gravis. Troubles in interpreting tests arise from the apparent increase in some muscles' strength during emotional stress, which most tests provoke.

— David B. Melchinger, M.D.
Associate Clinical Professor of Medicine,
Yale University School of Medicine

Arensberg, Ann. *Sister Wolf*. New York: Pocket Books, 1980.

Fox, Michael W. *The Soul of the Wolf*. Boston: Little, Brown and Company, 1980.

Frankl, Viktor E. *Man's Search for Meaning*. New York: Pocketbooks, Simon and Schuster, 1963.

Hesse, Hermann. *Steppenwolf*. New York: Bantam Books, 1980.

Kumin, Maxine. *To Make a Prairie*. Ann Arbor: University of Michigan Press, 1979.

Lopez, Barry Holstun. *Of Wolves and Men*. New York: Charles Scribner's Sons, 1978.

Mech, L. David. *The Wolf*. Minneapolis: University of Minnesota Press, 1970.

Mowat, Farley. *Never Cry Wolf*. Boston: Little, Brown and Company, 1963.

O'Connor, Flannery. *The Habit of Being*. New York: Farrar, Straus, and Giroux, 1979.

Register, Cheri. *Living with Chronic Illness*. New York: The Free Press, Macmillan, Inc., 1987.

Rollin, Betty. *Last Wish*. New York: Linden Press, 1985.

Rose, Phyllis. *Parrallel Lives*. New York: Alfred A. Knopf, 1984.

Strong, Maggie. *Mainstay: For the Spouse of the Chronically Ill*. Boston: Little, Brown and Company, 1988.

Turbak, Gary. *Twilight Hunters*. Flagstaff, Ariz.: Northland Press, 1987.